YUMMY CHEWING GUMS: TOXIC RIDDLE FOR THE TOXIC DETECTIVE

An Indian Society of Toxicology Initiative

Vivekanshu Verma

Vijay Vasudev Pillay

Shiv Rattan Kochar

Prateek Rastogi

Karen Harshita

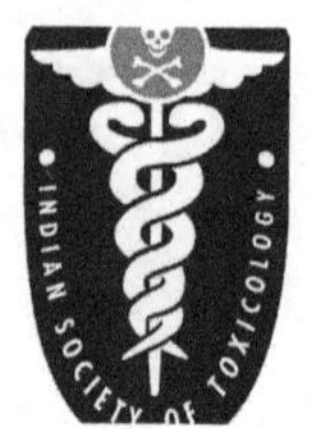

Dedicate the First Edition to……….
We dedicate this book on Toxic Riddles to all the Toxicology Nurses, Medical students, Senior residents, and fellows from the school of medicine, nursing, law, police academy and pharmacy, who strongly feel that Riddle solving approach is a must for all involved healthcare providers who strive to be the best caretakers of their patients suffering from poisoning, drug overdose or intoxication.
We hope that this book will aid all young budding toxicologists' quest to excellence, who want to practice their professional skills conscientiously and fearlessly and are keen to promote quality in healthcare of poisoning victims.
We are also grateful to our teachers, parents, elders and seniors for their blessings, constant motivation and support, in materializing the dream cum true of compiling a textbook on toxicology. We wish to dedicate this treatise to Late Dr Chiranji Lal Verma, who was an expert surgeon & guided in motivating us to become, what we,are today. In last, We would also dedicate this book to cute little niece Heeral, a bundle of joy, without whom, this would not have been possible.

CONTENTS

Yummy Chewing Gums: Toxic Riddle for the Toxic Detective

An Indian Society of Toxicology Initiative

Vivekanshu Verma
Vijay Vasudev Pillay
Shiv Rattan Kochar
Prateek Rastogi
Karen Harshita

PREFACE

Toxicology riddle solving is neither art
nor science, but rather a craft.

It requires a commitment to excellence from a craftsman.

Paying it forward is part of the deal.

This work is our attempt to share what we've learned
about Medical Toxicology with the next generation.

Writing a book is not an easy task, and neither
is being a Toxicologist.
Toxic Riddles narrated in Rhymes;
During Terror of Corona times;
By Toxic Detective for solving Crimes;
On Indian Society of Toxicology (IST)'s Paradigms;
Happy Learning!

Yummy Chewing Gums: Toxic Riddle for the Toxic Detective

An Indian Society of Toxicology Initiative

For Toxic Detectives, Crime Scene Investigators (CSi), Toxicologists, Police Officers, CID & CBI officers, Lawyers, Judges, Magistrates, Legal counsels, Law Students, Forensic Scientists, Doctors, Toxicology Nurses & Emergency Paramedics

Dr Vivekanshu Verma, MBBS, Postgraduate Diploma in Forensic Medicine & Toxicology, Fellow of Indian Society of Toxicology, Associate consultant, Emergency & Trauma care, Medanta-The Medicity, Gurugram. Honorary Toxicology Expert, Central Bureau of Investigation

Dr Vijay Vasudev Pillay, MBBS, MD Forensic Medicine & Toxicology, Chief, Poison Control Centre, Professor & Head, Forensic Medicine & Toxicology, Amrita School of Medicine, Amrita Vishwa Vidyapeetham, Cochin, Kerala

Dr Shiv Rattan Kochar, MBBS, MD Forensic Medicine & Toxicology, Senior Professor, Forensic Medicine. Chief Vigilance Officer, Metro MANAS Arogya Sadan Heart Care & Multispecialty Hospital, Directorate of Medical Education, Jaipur (Rajasthan)

Dr Prateek Rastogi, MBBS,MD, PGDMLE, PGDCFS, PGCMNCPA, PGCTM, Dip. Cyber Law, FAGE, FAIMER Fellow (MUFILIPE-Manipal), Former President, Indian Society of Toxicology(2018-19), Professor, Department of Forensic Medicine & Toxicology, Kasturba Medical College, Mangalore, Karnataka

Dr Karen Harshita, MD Forensic Medicine & Toxicology, Senior Resident, Forensic Medicine & Toxicology, Bangalore Medical College and research institute, Bangalore

©2021 Indian Society of Toxicology

Poison Control Centre

Amrita Institute of Medical Science,

Ponekkara, P. O, Kochi, Kerala - 682041.

ISBN:9798596618501

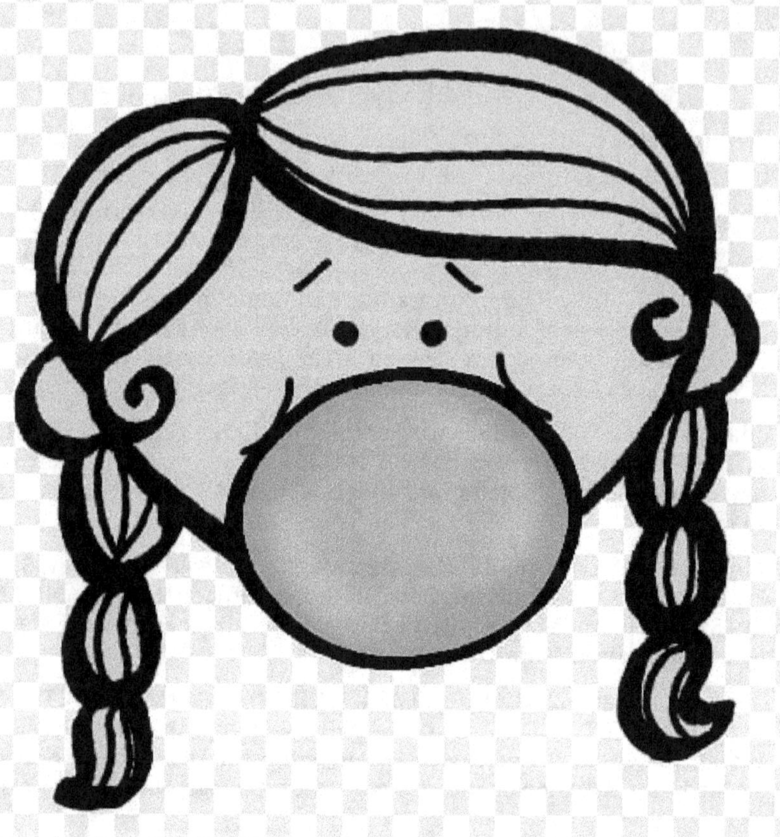

YUMMY CHEWING GUMS

209th Toxic Riddle in Rhymes to relieve covid's coughing bout

Let's solve an intoxicating riddle for "Gums to save Gums" sir

Its statuary warning- Don't misuse Zai Lee Tall & throw about

As if I was like a children's sugary bubble chewing gum to her

Teens chew my gum & blow bubble to show me in selfie pout

Masticating well, found me tasteless after enjoying my flavor

I Hold the Guinea's record as world's tallest angiosperm stout

Double mint center fresh Pink bubble you call Iipped us tweet

Blossomed, Petal-less, Closed Cupped flowers bloom in sprout

Fertile fluffy haired stamens scents cough lozenges
honey sweet

For venomous wasps & honeybees to buzz Spurious black about

Nilgiris tree bark make whitened Vicks
VapoRub on chest to meet

Koala bears gather Gum-nuts from us to sing a song through out

High Risk for kids to choke, if they slept & aspirate
gums they eat

May stuck the blue gumstick into airway instead
of spitting it out

Sugar gum leaves the Sigh a knighed, toxic to goats on four feet

The Giant gum trees of the UK lip tall centurion
standing in bout

My litter is lot in so huge & highly flammable to get on fired seat

I'm Australian forest fire hazard, bushfire mountain ash to snout

Rapid vaporization of my aroma oils results
in quick ignite to lit

The Swamp gum from my pointed leaves, sickle-shaped stout

But I have a saddest gum of sorrow, to share with all of u a bit,

I got so blamed by agree culture, for sucking soil's nutrients out

So banned to cultivate in India, by Hon'ble court's order to hit

2 0 9th Toxic Riddle in Rhymes to relieve covid's coughing bout
Let's solve an intoxicating campaign for "Gums to save Gums " sir
Its statuary warning- Don't misuse Zai Lee Tall & throw about
As if I was like a children's sugary bubble chewing gum to her
Teens chew my gum & blow balloon to show me in selfie pout
Masticating well, found me tasteless after enjoying my flavor
I Hold the Guinea's record as world's tallest angiosperm stout
Double mint center fresh Pink bubbled, you call lipped us tweet
Blossomed, Petal-less, Closed Cupped flowers bloom in sprout
Fertile fluffy haired stamens scents cough lozenges honey sweet
For Venomous wasps honeybees to buzz Spurious black about
Nilgiris bark & oil make whitened Vicks VapoRub on chest to meet
Koala Bears gather Gum nuts from us to sing a song through out
High Risk for kids to choke, if they slept & aspirate gums they eat
May stuck the blue gumstick into airway instead of spitting it out
Sugar gum leaves Sigh a knighed, toxic to goats on 4 feet
The Giant gum trees of the UK lip tall centurion standing in bout
My litter is lot in so huge & highly flammable to get on fired seat
I'm Australian forest fire hazard, bushfire mountain ash to snout
Rapid vaporization of my aroma oils results in quick ignite to lit
The Swamp gum from my pointed leaves, sickle-shaped stout
But I have a saddest gum of sorrow, to share with all of u a bit,
I got badly blamed by agree culture, for sucking soil's nutrients out
Got stay on, ban to cultivate in India, by Hon'ble court's order to hit

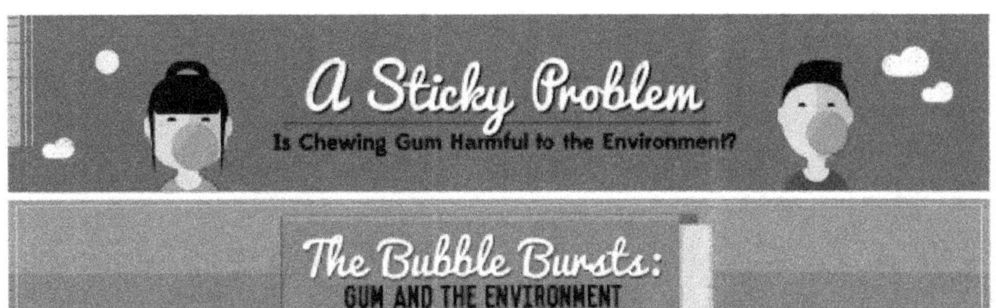

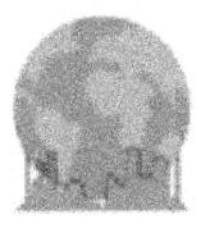

Though the consistency of gum is what makes it popular, it can lead to serious **environmental damage.**

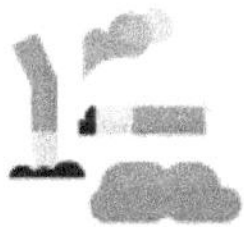

Chewing gum is the world's second most common form of litter after **cigarette butts.**

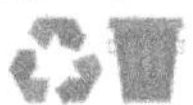

Disposal and collection of gum packaging at landfills costs more than $2 million annually.

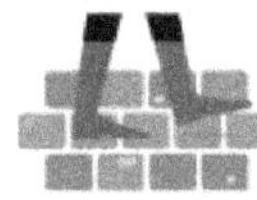

An estimated **92%** of Britain's urban paving stones have gum stuck to them.

CHEWING GUMS:

chewed with the gums

Gum is "resin from dried sap of plants," from Old French gome "(medicinal) gum, resin," from Late Latin gumma, from Latin gummi, from Greek kommi "gum," from Egyptian kemai.

As the name of a hardened, sweetened gelatine mixture as a candy.

Gum – What's in name ?

Gum has multiple meanings in different context:

• Gum in plants - chewing gums: Resin, look alike pink coloured gums.

• Gums in animals- tooth supported by pink fleshy gums: the tissue that surrounds the necks of teeth and covers the alveolar parts of the jaws.

• Gums in school- glue to stick (a substance or deposit resembling a plant gum, as in sticky or adhesive quality)

• Gum (ग़म) in hindi language means sorrow.

So what's the matter of ग़म (sorrow) with Gum:

•Litter of Chewing gums is 2nd highest in the world ranking, after the cigarette butts as 1st, as non-biodegradable health hazard.

•Litter of Gum tree, in form of dry leaves, is potentially hazardous, causing forest fire hazards, as its flammable, due to rich content of combustible oil.

• Its oil is aromatic & is popular rubefacient, but toxic on ingestion to kids & pets.

• Chewing Gums may stick in airway & cause choking in toddlers & pets, due to poor gag reflex

INTRODUCTION

Eucalyptus oil is a traditional remedy for a variety of common ailments, particularly of the respiratory tract.

It is cheap, freely available, and found in many households.

However, its extreme toxicity is not generally appreciated and reports of poisonings are rare.

With this in mind, we have compiled the reported cases of toxic ingestion of eucalyptus oil that was nearly fatal.

GUM TREE

When it comes to this magnificent genus of trees commonly called gum trees, there's a lot to know.

On the dullish end of the spectrum, we have facts about the word "eucalyptus".

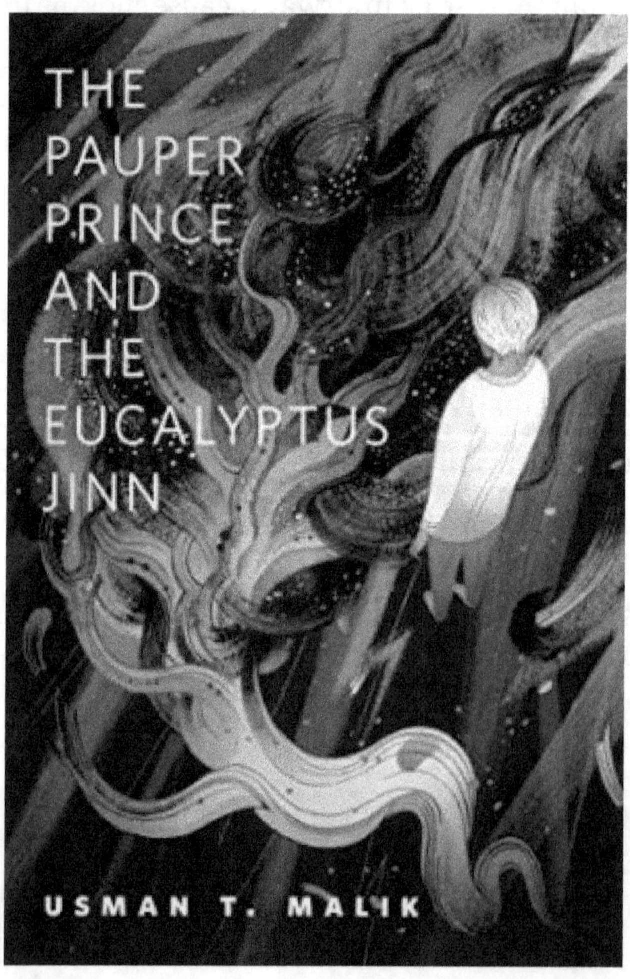

Figure 1. The Pauper Prince and the Eucalyptus Jinn. Malik Usman T (2015), A fictional Novel from Lahore Pakistan

WHAT DOES EUCALYPTUS MEAN?

It comes from a combination of Latin (EU meaning "from") and Greek (kalyptos meaning "covered" and kalyptein meaning "to conceal") used to describe the seed pod.

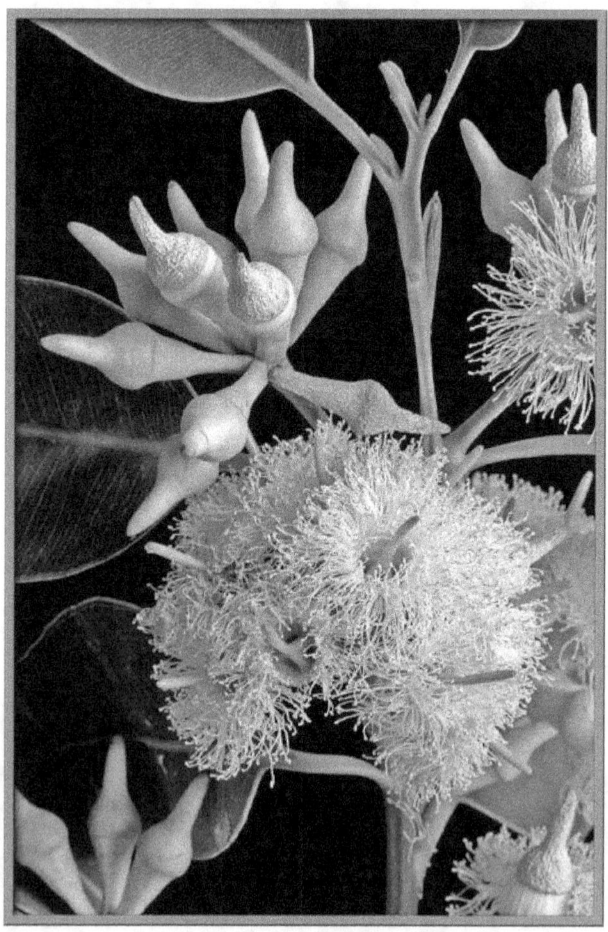

Figure 2. Eucalyptus flowers

The name eucalyptus comes from the Greek words 'eu' (beautiful) and 'kalyptos' (hat), because the stamens and pistils together resemble a hat.

GUM – WHAT'S IN NAME

Gum has multiple meanings in different context:

- Gum in plants - chewing gums: to chew with the gums
- Gums in animals- tooth supported by gums: the tissue that surrounds the necks of teeth and covers the alveolar parts of the jaws
- Gums in school- glue to stick (a substance or deposit resembling a plant gum, as in sticky or adhesive quality)
- Gum (ग़म) in hindi language means sorrow

Ref: https://www.merriam-webster.com/dictionary/gum

WHAT IS THE ROOT WORD FOR GUM?

gum (n.1) c. 1300, "resin from dried sap of plants," from Old French gome "(medicinal) gum, resin," from Late Latin gumma, from Latin gummi, from Greek kommi "gum," from Egyptian kemai.

As the name of a hardened, sweetened gelatine mixture as a candy.

WHY CHEWING GUMS NAMED SO?

chewing gums: to chew with the gums of the jaw in mouth. Gums in plants are any of numerous colloidal polysaccharide substances of plant origin that are gelatinous when moist but harden on drying and are salts of complex organic acids.

WHAT IS THE DIFFERENCE BETWEEN RESIN AND GUM?

Gums are viscous substances which are secreted by the bark of certain trees. ... Resins, on the other hand, are gluey and viscous substances which may be whiteish, brownish, or red and are secreted by certain trees when they are incised. Resins contain an essence and are usually not water soluble.

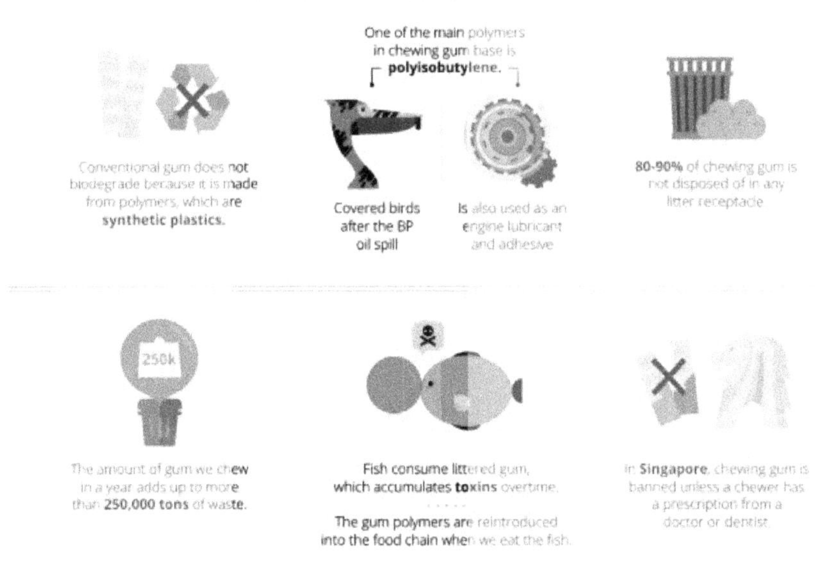

WHAT IS GUM MADE OF?

Gum base. Gum base is one of the main chewing gum ingredients found in gum and is made up of three main components: resin, wax and elastomer. In short, resin is the main chewable portion, whereas wax helps to soften the gum and elastomers help to add flexibility.

WHAT IS THE OLDEST GUM?

World's oldest piece of chewing gum is 5,000 years old. A 5,000-year-old piece of chewing gum, which was discovered by an archaeology student in Finland in 2007, is known as the oldest piece of chewing gum yet found.

GUM TREES

Eucalyptus trees are a diverse genus of flowering trees and shrubs in the myrtle family, known as Myrtaceae. Eucalyptus trees, which can come from either Eucalyptus, Corymbia, or Angophora genera, are sometimes called gum trees. This often suggests to people that the very gum they chew might come from these trees. Interestingly, some koala bears only eat a few varieties of these gum leaves, and many of its dried leaves and oil are popular uses of medicine.

DOES CHEWING GUM HELP JAWLINE?

Chewing gum is one of the easiest ways of improving your jawline definition. The chewing action works the muscles in your neck and jaw, which really tightens up the whole jawline and chin area. And if you're constantly chewing, you're working those muscles all day long

IS IT BAD TO SWALLOW GUM?

Although chewing gum is designed to be chewed and not swallowed, it generally isn't harmful if swallowed. ... If you swallow gum, it's true that your body can't digest it. But the gum doesn't stay in your stomach. It moves relatively intact through your digestive system and is excreted in your stool.

CAN A 3 YEAR OLD CHEW GUM?

It's okay to let your child enjoy a piece of gum every now and then, but the American Academy of Pediatrics recommends waiting until the child is old enough to understand not to swallow the gum.

WHAT HAPPENS IF 3 YEAR OLD SWALLOWED CHEWING GUM?

Chewing gum itself is not toxic or poisonous. * It is considered a foreign body. If 1 to 2 pieces are swallowed by a healthy child, no symptoms are expected. If a child has stomach or intestinal problems, more serious symptoms (such as blockage in the intestines) can occur.

CAN SWALLOWING GUM CAUSE A BLOCKAGE?

In rare cases, swallowing a large mass of gum, or many small pieces of gum over a short period of time, can block the digestive tract. Blockages are more likely to happen when gum is swallowed along with other indigestible things (like sunflower seed shells).

CAN SWALLOWING GUM HURT TODDLERS?

Although a swallowed piece of gum should pass through a child just as it would an adult, young children might swallow large quantities of gum and even objects that can get stuck to the gum in their digestive tract.

IS IT BAD TO SLEEP WITH GUM IN YOUR MOUTH?

You can choke or get a respiratory infection. You should just swallow it now. It could fall onto your sheets and get stuck.

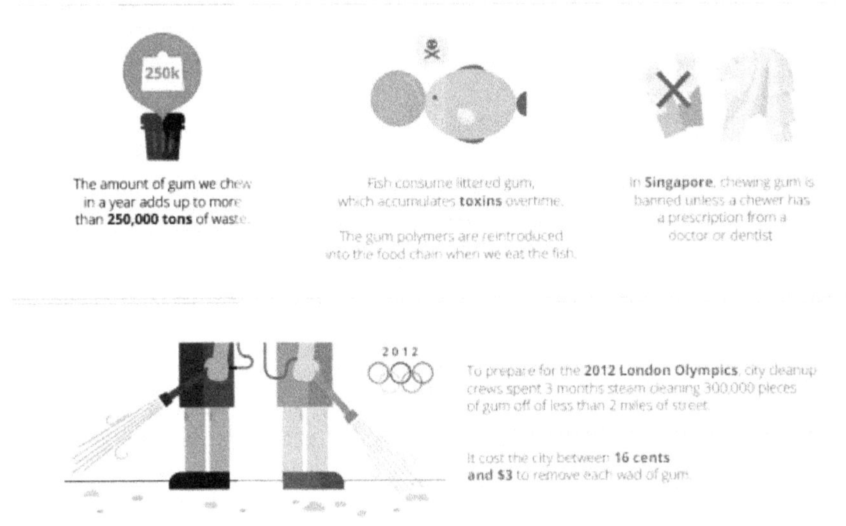

Figure 3. Chewing Gum. Image source: https://www.custommade.com/blog/content/uploads/2015/01/gum-final.jpg

CAN EXPIRED GUM KILL YOU?

According to the International Chewing Gum Association, chewing gum is very stable. This is because it's low in moisture and non-reactive. Gum is not required by law to have an expiration date in most countries because of this. ... While old gum may have a less desirable brittle texture, it's still safe to eat.

CAN CHEWING GUM MAKE YOU GAIN WEIGHT?

Chewing gum could make you FAT because the minty taste makes sugary food more tempting. It may well give you minty-fresh breath, but chewing gum could also cause weight gain, new research suggests. Scientists have discovered that people who chew gum eat more high calorie sweet foods.

IS SPITTING OUT GUM LITTERING?

80–90% of chewing gum is not disposed of properly and it's the second most common form of litter after cigarette butts.

Chewing gum is made from polymers which are synthetic plastics that do not biodegrade. ... These gums are natural, biodegradable substances.

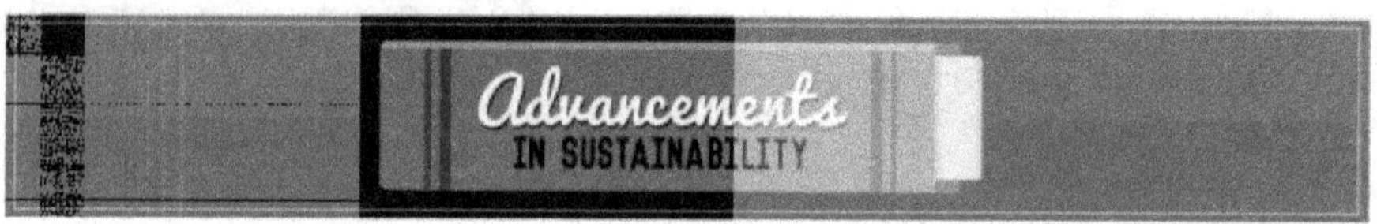

In 2011, a British scientist invented a sustainable alternative to chewing gum called **Rev7**.

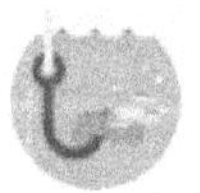

Unlike regular gum, which is water-resistant, this gum **dissolves** with water.

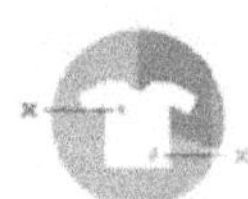

It's **30%** easier to remove from clothes and sidewalks.

With water and mild agitation, the gum can disintegrate into a **fine powder** in 6 months.

There are also modern-day **chicle-based** gums that biodegrade completely in 2 weeks.

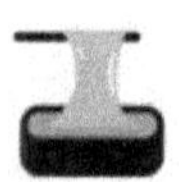

Chicle is a natural form of rubber.

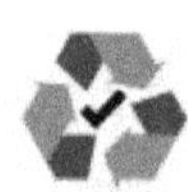

It's **100% biodegradeable.**

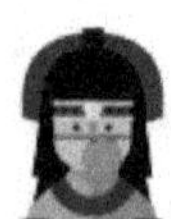

The gum we chew now is meant to mimic the chicle-based gum the **ancient Mayans** chewed.

IS THERE A NATURAL CHEWING GUM?

Functional Gums has launched Natur Gum, which it claims is the first 100% natural chewing gum, made of 100% biodegradable and natural gum base. Natur Gum only contains natural flavorings and natural sweeteners such as stevia or xylitol for consumers who want natural products and eco-friendly choices.

WHAT TREE DOES GUM COME FROM?

Chicle or Naseberry (Manilkara zapota), a native tree of Central America and the West Indies. The fruit is also known as the sapodilla. The fleshy pulp is used to make sapodilla custard and ice cream. Chicle gum is extracted from the sap of the trunk and is used in some natural chewing gums to this day.

WHICH PLANT GIVES US GUM?

Gum Acacia

Gum arabic is the most widely used of the water-soluble gums.

True gum arabic is gum acacia; that is, it is produced by species of Acacia.

WHAT IS ANOTHER NAME FOR GUM TREES?

12 Species of Gum Trees. Within the myrtle (Myrtaceae) family of plants, there are three genera containing shrub and tree species commonly known as gum trees: Eucalyptus (the majority of gum species), Angophora, and Corymbia.

CHEWING GUM & GUM TREES

Natural chewing gum from trees does not widely occur today, partially because it's unsustainable to harvest. This also leads to environmental issues, as trees die off, contributing to forest depletion. Rather than killing off our trees, chewing gum manufacturers have been using synthetic bases since the 1980s. According to the Gum Companies claims, modern gums are made with chicle, natural gums, or human-made latex. Other human-made materials are added for a better chewing experience. While modern commercial brands of gum does not come from the gum trees, you could try chewing Eucalyptus resin when you find one of these trees.

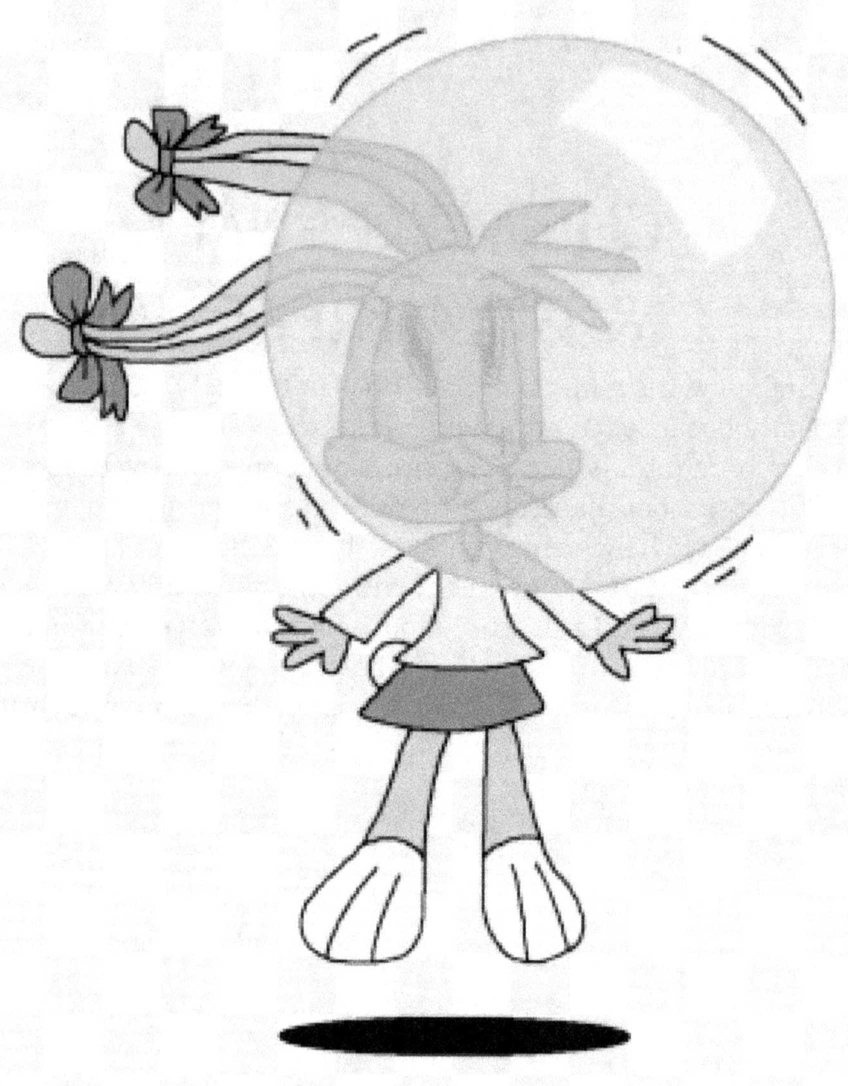

WOOD'S BLOOD
- RED GUM

There is Kino, which is the name of plant gum produced by plants and trees including Eucalyptus.

It produces a red color that oozes out large amounts, where it gets its name "red gum" and "blood wood."

This type of gum is used in medicine, tanning, and dyes, but not as chewing gum.

However, it was used as a traditional remedy for issues with diarrhea and sore throats.

Myers, Vanessa Richins. "Natural Chewing Gum History and Facts." ThoughtCo, Sep. 23, 2020, thoughtco.com/does-chewing-gum-come-from-gum-trees-3269782.

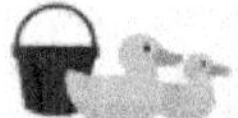

What to do with
ALREADY-BEEN-CHEWED GUM

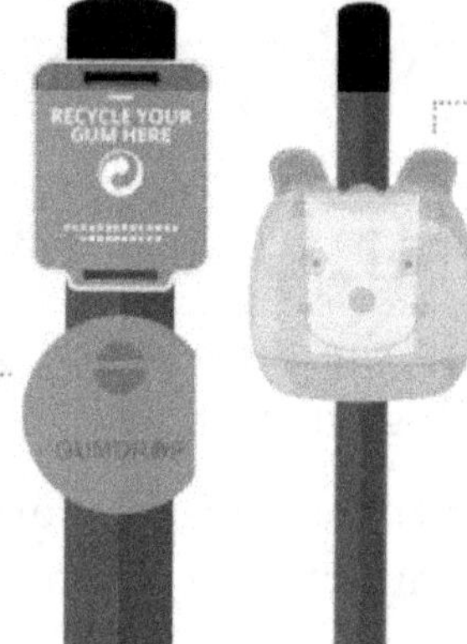

Inventors developed a technology to recycle chewed gum (which can be turned into **rubber containers or children's toys**).

This technology requires chewers to throw used gum into **specially designated waste containers**.

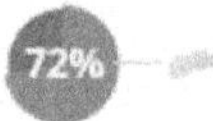

········ Similarly, the **Gummy Bin** helps reduce chewing gum litter.

72%

It reduced chewing gum litter by **72%** over a six-month period in 2006.

The recycled gum can be turned into **drainage and construction material**.

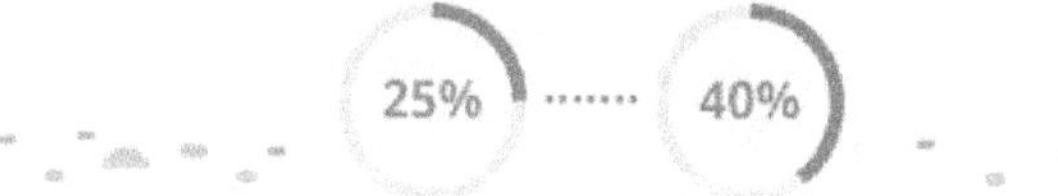

The UK's Chewing Gum Action Group (CGAC) have reduced littered gum by as much as 25–40% by promoting good disposal practice through:

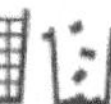
On-pack icons

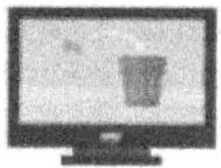
Proper disposal messages in advertising and at point of sale

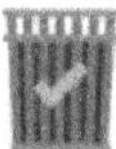
Where specified gum bins are not available, the next best option is to wrap chewed gum and place it in a trash can.

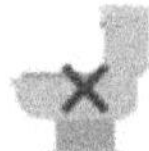
Do not flush it down the **toilet** or throw it into **waterways**.

The truth of the matter is, gum isn't going anywhere. The demand is high, but so is gum's lasting power in the environment.
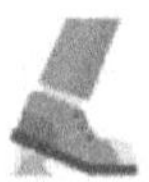

WHAT IS THE COMMON EUCALYPTUS?

Eucalyptus globulus, commonly known as southern blue gum, is a species of tall, evergreen tree endemic to southeastern Australia.

EUCALYPTUS GLOBULUS

Family = Myrtaceae.

Habitat = Native to Australia; now cultivated mainly at the hill-stations of India.

English Blue-Gum tree, Australian Gum tree.

Ayurvedic Tilaparna, Tailaparna, Sugandhapatra, Haritaparna Neelaniryaasa, Tribhandi, Triputaa, Saralaa, Suvahaa, Rechani, Nishotraa.

Unani = Neelgiri oil.

Siddha/Tamil = Karpooramaram.

ACTION

Essential oil from leaves— antiseptic, antibiotic, antiviral, antifungal, antispasmodic, decongestant, antiasthmatic, expectorant, antirheumatic, diaphoretic.

Used in chronic, bronchitis, migraine, congestive headache, neuralgia and ague, as an inhalant or internal medicine.

Root—purgative.

KEY APPLICATION

Leaf tea for catarrhs of the respiratory tract.

Oil used externally for rheumatic complaints, contraindicated internally in inflammatory diseases of the gastrointestinal tract, bile ducts, and in severe liver diseases.

Its Oil—as adjuvant treatment of chronic obstructive respiratory complaints, including bronchitis and bronchial asthma, also for symptomatic relief of colds and catarrh of the upper respiratory tract; externally for symptomatic treatment of colds and rheumatic complaints.

Leaf—antiseptic.

E. globulus is the main commercial source of Eucalyptus leaf oil; yield is 2.12%; 1,8-cineole exceeds 70% (pharmaceutical grade oil requires a minimum cineole content of 70%).

Several potent euglobals, having closely related acyl-phloroglucinolmonoterpene (or sesquiterpene) structures, are isolated from the leaves and flower buds.

These compounds showed strong granulation-inhibiting activity and inhibition of TPA induced EBV (Epstein-Barr Virus) activation.

Phloroglucin derivatives, isolated from leaves, showed better anti-inflammatory activity than indomethacin.

Natural antioxidants have also been isolated from the plant.

Dosage of Leaf decoction = 50–100 ml for inhalation.

Khare, CP. Indian Medicinal Plants: An Illustrated Dictionary. Springer. 2007. Eucalyptus p247.

IS EUCALYPTUS OIL SAFE TO INHALE?

Eucalyptus is used for its soothing effects when inhaled, for example during a cold or cough.

The toxic effects of eucalyptus oil alone include a burning sensation in the mouth and throat, spontaneous vomiting, respiratory difficulty and CNS depression progressing to seizures.

WHY ITS SO POPULAR?

Essential oils are volatile oils that have been used for centuries as topical rubefacients, analgesics and antipyretics.

They are found in many over-the-counter remedies, and are inexpensive and widely used in the treatment of coughs due to colds.

The essential oil products frequently encountered in poisonings are camphorated oil (20% camphor), eucalyptus oil (70%) or a combination in Vicks VaporRub (Procter & Gamble, Canada) ointment (4.3% camphor, 6% eucalyptus oil, 4% menthol), VapAir (Drug Trading, Canada) vaporizing liquid (2% camphor, 6% eucalyptus oil, 4% menthol) and Camphor-Phenique (Bayer Corporation, USA) (10.8% camphor, 4.7% phenol).

Parents and caregivers may not be aware of the potentially toxic effects of these oils and products if they are ingested orally by an infant or a child.

Flaman, Z et al. "Unintentional exposure of young children to camphor and eucalyptus oils." Paediatrics & child health vol. 6,2 (2001): 80-3. doi:10.1093/pch/6.2.80

HOW MUCH EUCALYPTUS IS TOXIC?

Dose related toxicity: Even small ingestions of pure oil can lead to severe symptoms.

In a dose of 2-3 mL; can expect mild CNS depression with drowsiness and/or dizziness and ataxia.

In a dose of ≥5 mL can expect significant CNS depression with coma.

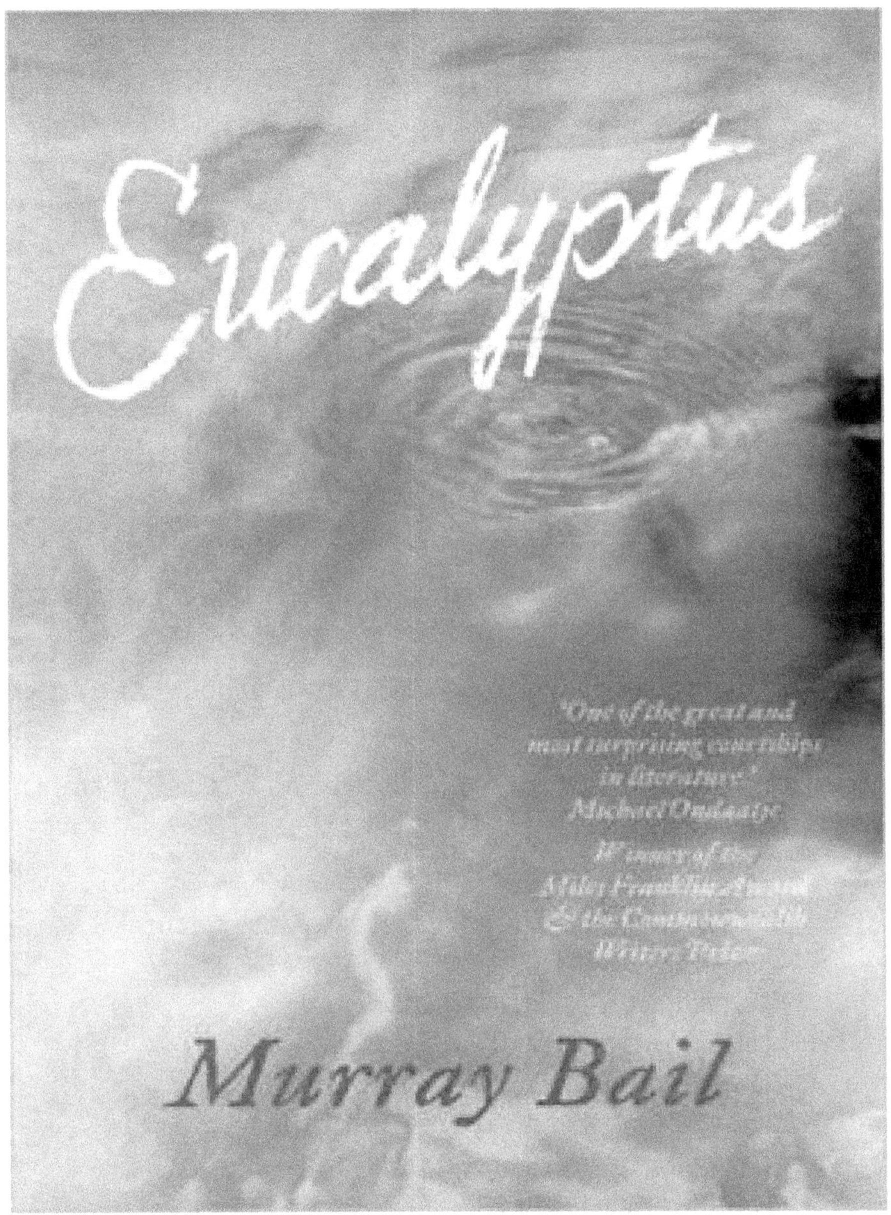

Figure 4. Eucalyptus. Bail Murray (2010), A Novel

WHAT ARE TOXIC EFFECTS ASSOCIATED WITH SWALLOWING EUCALYPTUS OIL?

The clinical effects of eucalyptus oil preparations are epigastric pain, vomiting and CNS symptoms.

CNS symptoms can develop within 30 min, although the onset may be delayed for up to 4 h.

Ingestion of 3 to 5 mL of pure eucalyptus oil has caused transient coma and even seizures.

- If swallowed, eucalyptus oil can cause seizures,
- Abdominal pain.
- Blue discoloration of skin.
- Shortness of breath.
- Problems with coordination.
- Low blood pressure (hypotension)
- Irregular heart beats (arrhythmias)
- Multi-organ failure.

WHICH EUCALYPTUS OIL IS BEST?

Blue Mallee (Eucalyptus polybractea).

Blue Mallee oil is the strongest Eucalyptus essential oil with extremely high eucalyptol content.

This makes the oil powerfully therapeutic but also most in need of dilution before use.

EUCALYPTOL

Eucalyptus Oil is the oil extracted from the leaves of various Eucalyptus species.

Oxides: Eucalyptol is an oxide volatile oil found in the Eucalyptus Tree.

Eucalyptus oil is used for its aromatic properties and as an ingredient in pharmaceutical and industrial applications.

Eucalyptol is an ingredient in many brands of mouthwash and cough suppressant.

It controls airway mucus hypersecretion and asthma via anti-inflammatory cytokine inhibition.

Eucalyptol is an effective treatment for nonpurulent rhinosinusitis.

Eucalyptol reduces inflammation and pain when applied topically.

Steyn DG (1948) The toxicity of various species of Eucalyptus trees (blue gum, blougom, bloekom). J S Afr Vet Assoc 19(Mar):25-29.

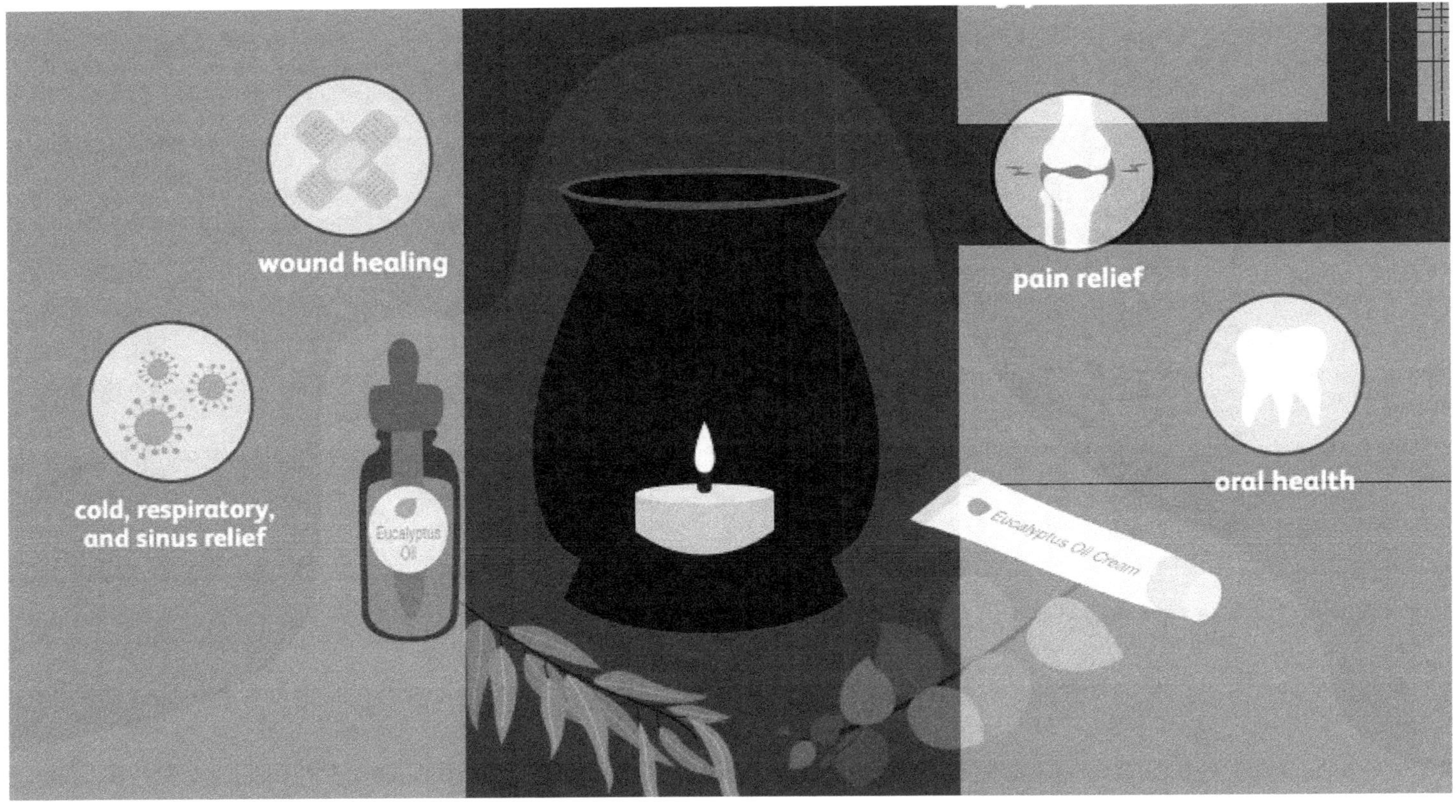

wound healing
cold, respiratory, and sinus relief
Eucalyptus Oil
pain relief
oral health
Eucalyptus Oil Cream

WHAT IS NILGIRI FAMOUS FOR?

Nilgiris is known for its eucalyptus oil and tea, and also produces bauxite. Some tourists are attracted to study the lifestyles of the various tribes living here or to visit the tea and vegetable plantations.

DOES EUCALYPTUS OIL KILL VIRUS?

In one lab study, it outperformed the standard herpes medication, acyclovir. The 1,8-cineole chemical in the oil shuts down virus particles and may block them from entering cells. In lab tests, eucalyptus oil was able to curb the spread of the virus by more than 96%.

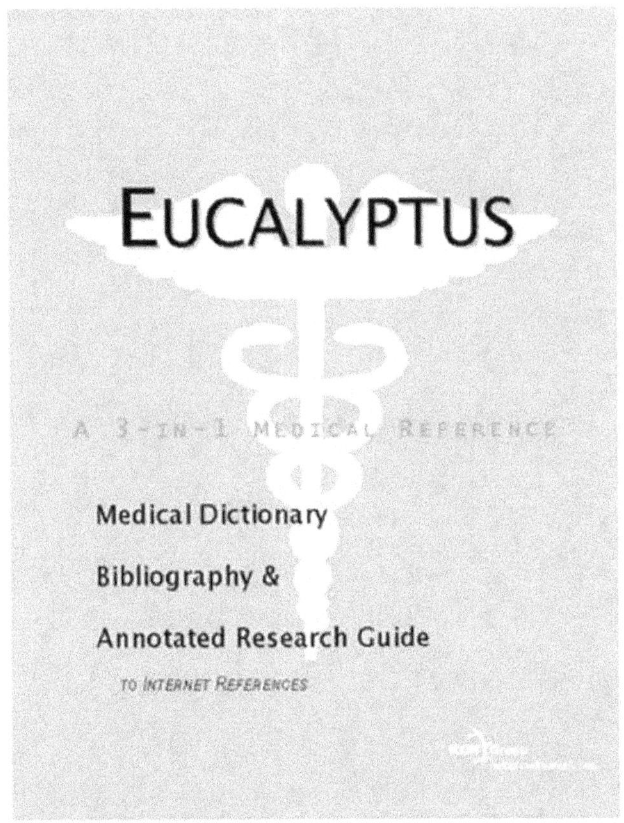

Figure 5.Eucalyptus - A Medical Dictionary, Bibliography, and Annotated Research Guide to Internet References (2004)

IS EUCALYPTUS BAD FOR ENVIRONMENT?

One of the biggest problems with eucalyptus trees is their negative impact on the environment. They have replaced indigenous forests in several parts of the world, depleting food and shelter sources and therefore affecting animals and birds. ... The natural oils of the eucalyptus tree make it extremely flammable.

ARE EUCALYPTUS TREES DANGEROUS?

Blue gum eucalyptus is one of the most fire-intensive plants. Trees not only put a lot of fuel on the ground as they shed bark, leaves and twigs, but in intense fires, volatile compounds in foliage cause explosive burning.

DO EUCALYPTUS TREES EXPLODE?

Eucalypts can indeed explode; in the heat of a fire, the sap of the tree expands and can seep through cracks in the bark. ... Instead, what can happen - and indeed, leads many Australian bushfires to spread so widely - is that sparks can be blown across several miles, igniting new 'spot' fires some distance away.

RIDDLE ANALYSIS

209TH TOXIC RIDDLE IN RHYMES TO RELIEVE COVID'S COUGHING BOUT

Owing to their lipophilic nature, Essential Oils (EOs) of Eucalyptus are advocated to penetrate viral membranes easily leading to membrane disruption.

Moreover, EOs contain multiple active phytochemicals that can act synergistically on multiple stages of viral replication and also induce positive effects on host respiratory system including bronchodilation and mucus lysis.

At present, only computer-aided docking and few in vitro studies are available which show anti-SARC-CoV-2 activities of EOs.

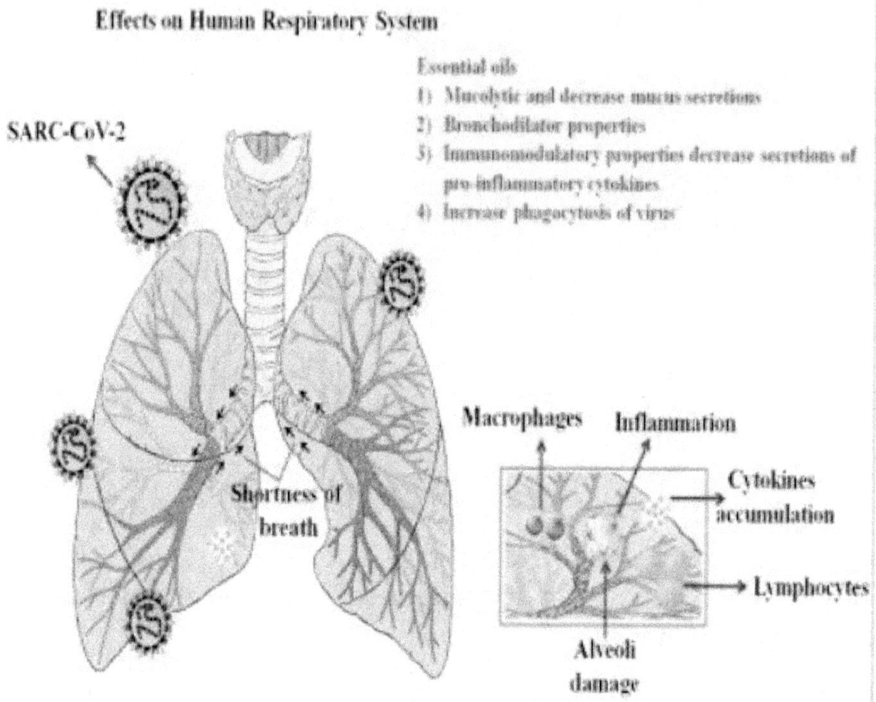

Figure 7. Eucalyptus oil helps in curing corona infection. Image source: Asif, Muhammad et al. "COVID-19 and therapy with essential oils having antiviral, anti-inflammatory, and immunomodulatory properties." Inflammopharmacology vol. 28,5 (2020): 1153-1161. doi:10.1007/s10787-020-00744-0

THE GIANT GUM TREES OF THE UK LIP TALL CENTURION STANDING IN BOUT

UK-Lip – Tall = Eu-ca-lyp-tol = Eucalyptol

Many of the world's most impressive trees have grand names, but Centurion's came about by coincidence. Rather than being named for its towering 100m height, the name was reserved for the 100th monumental tree recorded as part of a wider Tasmanian tree-measuring project.

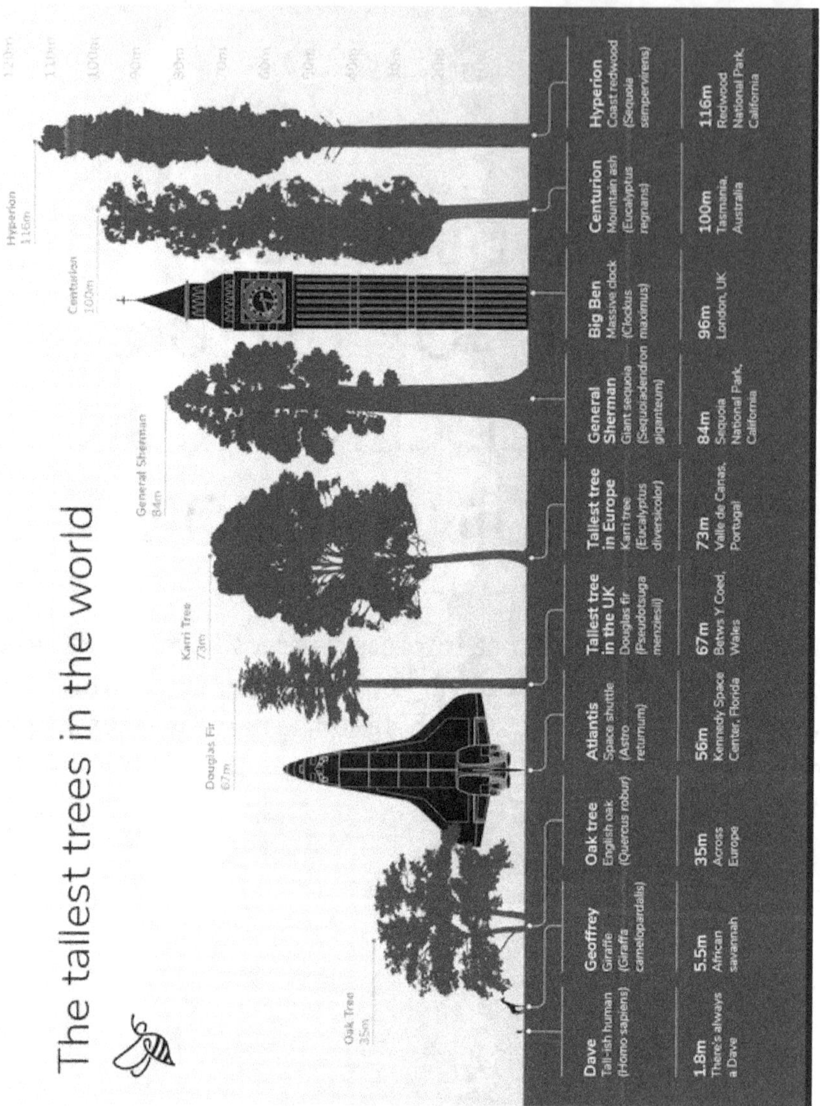

Figure 6. The Tallest Trees in the World. Image source: https://medium.com/@candidegardening/the-tallest-trees-in-the-world

As redwoods are technically softwood trees (defined by their seeds rather than the actual hardness of the wood), Centurion also holds the honour of being the world's tallest hardwood tree. And it was probably even taller in the past. Signs of a broken branch near the top of the tree suggest that Centurion could grow even higher in future.

Another magnificently named goliath, Centurion is a mountain ash (Eucalyptus regnans aka swamp gum) located in the untamed wilds of Tasmania. Having grown 80cm since its previous official measurement a few years before, in 2018 Centurion was measured at an incredible 100.5m. At the time, that made it the only known tree taller than 100m outside of North America.

ORIGIN OF SUBSTANCE

Eucalyptus oil is obtained by tesifying the oil distilled from leaves of various species of Eucalyptus.

The major active ingredient is cineole (eucalyptol).

- Its Colorless to pale yellow liquid.
- Odour: Camphoraceous odour
- Taste: Pungent, spicy, cooling taste
- Solubility: Insoluble in water
- Soluble 1 in 5 of alcohol 70%, Miscible with alcohol (90%), dehydrated alcohol, oils, fats and paraffins
- Miscible with ether, chloroform, glacial acetic acid.
- Boiling point of cineole (eucalyptol): 176°C to 177°C.
- Density of cineole (eucalyptol) 0.921 to 0.923
- Eucalyptus oil contains not less than 70 % W/W of cineole; it also contains pinene and other terpenes and may contain small quantities of phellandrene.
- Depending on the source -and purity- up to 41 compounds have been detected in eucalyptus oil the main component being cineole.

CHEMICAL NAME OF EUCALYPTOL:

- 1,3,3-Trimethyl-2-oxabicyclo[2.2.2.]-octane

Other chemical names: 1,8-epoxy-p-menthane

- Molecular formula of cineole (eucalyptol): C10H18O
- Molecular weight: 154.25.

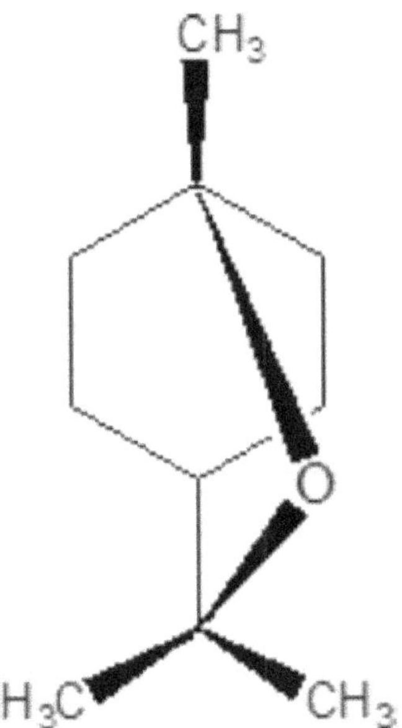

Structure of eucalyptol (1, 3, 3-Trimethyl-2-oxabicyclo [2. 2. 2]octane)

MEDICINAL

Eucalyptus oil has been used for inhalation as a decongestant often in combination with other volatile substances.

It has been used orally for catarrh and coughs.

It has been applied as a rubefacient.

It has been used as a flavouring.

It is used extensively as a cleaning solvent.

It is used extensively as a fragrance.

It is used as an antiseptic, febrifuge and expectorant in herbal medicine.

STORAGE CONDITIONS

- Products containing eucalyptus oil should be stored at a temperature not exceeding 25 °C in well filled containers.
- Protect from light
- Liquid products containing eucalyptus oil are best stored in child resistant containers.

THERAPEUTIC DOSAGE

In Adults, Recommended adult oral dose is 0.05 mL to 0.2 mL
Has been used as a topical rubefacient at 0.5% to 3%.

Children=There is no recommended oral paediatric dose.

ROUTES OF ENTRY

1) Oral= Well absorbed orally.

Absorption expected to increase in the presence of lipid substances such as milk.

Gastrointestinal absorption is rapid.

It is lipid soluble and absorption is likely to be enhanced with foods such as milk.

2) Inhalation= Inhalation of the liquid or aerosol can be directly toxic to the lungs.

Citation: Owen FJ (1885) Notes on a case of poisoning by eucalyptus. Med J Aust, Sept 15: 394-397.

TOXICOKINETICS

Administration of 200 mg/kg of eucalyptol p.o. to rabbits showed peak plasma concentrations of the alicyclic substance, eucalyptol and its major unconjugated metabolites occurred within 30 min and 1 hour.

The Parent ether reached Cmax of 840 µg/dl within 30 min, while the plasma concentration of the chief unconjugated metabolite, (+)-2-exo-hydroxy-1, 8-cineole, peaked at 2400 µg/dl within 1 h and then decreased slowly between 2 hour and 6 hour.

Peak plasma concentration (1250 µg/dl) of the major conjugated metabolite, (+)-2-exo-hydroxy- 1,8-cineole, occurred 1.5–2 h after dosing.

Miyazawa M, Shindo M. Biotransformation of 1, 8-cineole by human liver microsomes, Nat. Prod. Lett. 2001;15(1):49-53.

METABOLIC RATE

In mice, 4 µl, 20 µl or 40 µl of rosemary oil containing 39% of eucalyptol (approximately equivalent to 52, 260 and 520 mg/kg of eucalyptol, respectively) is given by oral route shows blood concentrations of eucalyptol reached a peak 5 min.

At 260 mg/kg, blood concentrations remained constant over the next 90 min, while at 520 mg/kg, the peak blood concentration dropped to 60% of the maximum value and remained in that range for the following 80 min.

These results indicate that at doses of up to 200 mg/kg, eucalyptol goes through a rapid absorption into the blood, metabolism and conjugation to polar metabolites. At higher or inflated doses, however, metabolism appears to be slow, probably due to saturation of the metabolic pathway.

Kovar KA, Gropper B, Friess D, Ammon HPT. Blood levels of 1, 8-cineole and locomotor activity of mice after inhalation and oral administration of rosemary oil. Planta Medica. 1987;53(4):315-18

MILK & EUCALYPTOL

Eucalyptol is quickly absorbed from the gastrointestinal tract.

It's lipid soluble and absorption is enhanced in the presence of milk.

Inhalation of the liquid is directly toxic to the lungs

ELIMINATION AND EXCRETION

It is excreted via the lungs, urine, skin and faeces.

Eucalyptol undergoes oxidation in vivo with the formation of hydroxycineole which excretes as glucuronide.

Citation: MacPherson J (1925) The toxicology of eucalyptus oil. Med J Aust, 2: 108-110.

FATAL DOSE

Probable lethal dose of eucalyptol =0.05 mL to 0.5mL/kg

Ref: Hindle RC (1994) Eucalyptus oil ingestion. N Z Med J, May: 185-186.

LD50 (ORAL)

LD50 (ORAL) rat of cineole (Eucalyptol) 2480 mg/kg.

Citation: Jenner PM, Hagan EC, Taylor JM, Cook EL & Fitzhugh OG (1964) Food flavourings and compounds of related structure. Fd Cosmet Toxicol, 2: 327-343.

CAUTION

The use of eucalyptol containing products in children below 30 months old should be avoided.

Children younger than 7 years, the eucalyptol content of the finished product should not exceed 1.12% and its presence should be mentioned in the product labelling.

INGESTION

Tibballs (1995) observed that Poisoning affects the central nervous system (loss of consciousness, hypoventilation, depression of reflexes and convulsions), the gastrointestinal system (abdominal pain, vomiting and diarrhoea) and the respiratory system (respiratory depression, dyspnoea, pneumonitis and bronchospasm)

Citation: Tibballs J (1995) Clinical effects and management of eucalyptus oil ingestion in infants and young children. Med J Aust, 163: 177-180.

GIT TOXICITY

Gastrointestinal effects are frequently the initial effects (Foggie, 1911) although drowsiness may occur in a few minutes and coma within 10 minutes.

Foggie WE (1911) Eucalyptus oil poisoning. Br Med J, 1: 359-360.

HEPATOTOXICITY

An increase in liver enzyme activity was also found in mice given 500 mg/kg bw orally.

Single subcutaneous doses of 250 or 500 mg/kg bw increased the activity of drug metabolizing enzymes and stimulated bile flow.

NEUROTOXICITY-METABOLIC ENCEPHALOPATHY

The patient may vomit while drowsy or unconscious and aspiration is a major risk.

Craig JD (1953) Poisoning by the volatile oils in childhood. Arch Dis Child, 28: 475-483.

CARDIOTOXICITY

Tachycardia and weak irregular pulse has been noted (Kirkness, 1910).

Kirkness WR (1910) Poisoning by oil of eucalyptus. Br Med J, 1: 261.

Muscle weakness and ataxia may occur (MacPherson, 1925).

Nephritis is rare but has been

recorded (Gurr & Scroggie, 1965). Both miosis and mydriasis can occur(miosis being more common) (Webb &

Pitt, 1993). CNS depression or vomiting have been

delayed up to four hours (Wood, 1900; Foggie, 1911).

Recovery is often within 24 hours.

INHALATION

Inhalation of eucalyptus oil either as liquid

or aerosol may result in pneumonitis
(Krueger, 1967).

Krueger RP (1967) Chemical pneumonitis from
medicated vapour aerosol spraying. Clin Ped, Aug: 465-467.

Inhalation of vapour may
be used medicinally and there

is no data available on toxicity by this route

(Tibballs & James, 1995). Tibballs J &
James A (1995) Eucalyptus oil-medicinal therapy or
folk remedy? Aust J Hosp
Pharm, 25(6): 516-519.

CARCINOGENICITY

Eucalyptus oil appeared to have weak tumour promoting activity on mouse skin.

Citation: Roe FJC & Field WEH (1965) Chronic toxicity of essential oils and certain other products of natural origin. Fd Cosmet Toxicol, 3: 331-324

TOXICITY IN CHILDREN

Although many children remain asymptomatic after ingestions clinically significant symptoms have been reported following ingestion of less than one teaspoonful.

Citation: Craig JD (1953) Poisoning by the volatile oils in childhood. Arch Dis Child, 28: 475-483.

TOXICITY IN INFANTS

Anticipate minor depression of consciousness after ingestion of 2 mL to 3mL of pure eucalyptus oil and significant depression after more than 5 mL.

Citation: Tibballs J (1995) Clinical effects and management of eucalyptus oil ingestion in infants and young children. Med J Aust, 163: 177-180.

Severe poisoning has occurred after ingestion of 4 mL to 5 mL.

Citation: Foggie WE (1911) Eucalyptus oil poisoning. Br Med J, 1: 359-360.

KID'S TOXIC CASE

A boy of 6, who had occasionally been in the habit of getting a drop or two of eucalyptus oil on sugar, was given by mistaken a teaspoonful of the same.

This was about 6 o'clock one evening.

About 8 he had his usual light supper, and within two hours thereafter abdominal pain and severe vomiting sets in.

The vomiting continued without cessation of any length and diarrhoea soon became marked.

By 11 o'clock the boy became drowsy, and when he was seen about this time he was semi-comatose.

He was pale and collapsed, with a small but not very quick pulse.

The muscles generally were flaccid. The' pupils were medium in size and equal.

The conjunctival reflex was not quite abolished. The tendon reflexes were present and were not exaggerated.

There was no cough and the breathing was shallow. He could be roused by very vigorous slapping of the face, but each time he looked dazed. Every time he was awakened up the sickness and vomiting set in.

The vomited matter, which consisted of mucus and watery material, had a strong smell of eucalyptus oil.

After two or three hours of external stimulation very much along the lines usually adopted for opium poisoning, the heavy comatose condition appeared to pass off, and the child was allowed to sleep.

He slept well and next morning, beyond being a little tired, was quite himself again.

The breath had a smell of eucalyptus oil for three days.

There was never any irritation of the urinary tract. In brief, the poison showed itself by gastro-intestinal irritation and cerebral paresis.

Allan J (1910) Poisoning by oil of eucalyptus. Br Med J, 1: 569.

TODDLER'S CASE

In 1901, Benjamin et al. reported a toddler aged 2 years and 9 months, who had swallowed 2 drachma

of eucalyptus oil.

He was unconscious, and collapsed, with a quick pulse, stertorous breathing, and pupils contracted almost to a pin-point, just as in opium poisoning.

This pupil contraction, indeed, was the most striking feature in the symptoms.

The child had vomited immediately after taking the oil, and purging quickly set in.

CASE OF RECOVERY AFTER GASTRIC LAVAGE

Accidental ingestion of eucalyptus oil by a 3-year-old boy caused profound central nervous system depression within 30 minutes, but he recovered rapidly after gastric lavage.

Case facts: A 3-year-old boy was seen within 30 minutes of ingesting about 10 ml eucalyptus oil.

On examination he was deeply comatose and his breath smelt strongly of eucalyptus.

The pupils were constricted, muscle tone was markedly reduced, and his tendon reflexes could not be elicited.

His respirations were shallow and irregular at a rate of 10/min.

The pulse rate was 70 beats/min and the blood pressure 75/40 mmHg.

Biochemical investigations on admission included a serum urea of 6 3 mmol/l (38 mg/100 ml), with normal electrolytes.

Initial treatment included the insertion of a cuffed endotracheal tube (which produced no gag reflex), and gastric lavage with sodium bicarbonate solution.

Sodium sulphate 100 ml was left in the stomach as a cathartic.

By 2 hours after admission his pulse, blood pressure, and respiration rate had gradually returned to normal.

After 5 hours consciousness had gradually been regained, and by 24 hours physical examination was normal apart from a faint smell of eucalyptus on the breath.

Urinary output remained satisfactory throughout. He was discharged home 48 hours after admission.

Patel S & Wiggins J (1980) Eucalyptus oil poisoning. Arch Dis Child, 55: 405-406.

MAIN RISKS AND TARGET ORGANS

The main risk is aspiration secondary to vomiting and loss of consciousness.

Target organs are the central nervous system, the lungs and the gastrointestinal system.

Benjamin J (1906) Eucalyptus poisoning. Br Med J, 1: 1020.

SUMMARY OF CLINICAL EFFECTS

Poisoning affects the nervous system (loss of consciousness, hypoventilation, depression of reflexes and
convulsions), the gastrointestinal system (abdominal pain, vomiting and diarrhoea) and the respiratory system (respiratory depression, dyspnoea, pneumonitis and bronchospasm).

Gastrointestinal effects are frequently the initial effects although drowsiness may occur in a few
minutes and coma within 10 minutes. The patient may vomit while drowsy or unconscious and aspiration is a major risk.

Tachycardia and weak irregular pulse has been noted.
Muscle weakness and ataxia may occur.
Nephritis is rare but has been recorded.
Both miosis and mydriasis can occur (miosis being more common).
Central nervous system (CNS) depression or vomiting have been delayed up to four hours.
Recovery is often within 24 hours.

It is a mild skin irritant.

Chronic effects have not been reported.

DIAGNOSIS

In the absence of a relevant history the odour of eucalyptus should help make the diagnosis succinct. The breath, vomit and urine may all smell of eucalyptus.

DECONTAMINATION

Emesis is contraindicated.

Activated charcoal is indicated if the patient is unconscious or a large ingestion is suspected. Aspiration of eucalyptus and/or charcoal is a major risk. Therefore careful gastric lavage and instillation of activated charcoal or colonic washout solution should only be attempted under general anaesthesia with endotracheal intubation.

The role of catharsis has not been adequately assessed.

ENHANCED ELIMINATION

No data available. However, although peritoneal and hemodialysis has been reported for the management of eucalyptus oil ingestion- its routine use has not been established.

ILLUSTRATIVE CASES

Case reports from the literature

1) In 1905, Taylor reported that, after evening supper an adult male took a large teaspoonful of eucalyptus oil. He immediately experienced oesophageal pain followed by gasping for breath, restlessness, convulsive movements of his hands and was semicomatose passing to coma.

Vomiting was induced prior to him becoming comatose and he gradually recovered consciousness being quite well by next morning.

Case Citation: Taylor HS (1905) A case of acute poisoning by eucalyptus oil. Lancet, 2: 963-964.

2) In 1910, Kirkness reported that, an adult male who took 10 mL to 15 mL of eucalyptus oil became ataxic and faint within ten minutes.

He soon had distressing dyspnoea, weak pulse and violent vomiting.

His skin was greenish-yellow.

Half an hour after ingestion he was very drowsy, had painful and excessive micturition and was experiencing violent diarrhoea.

For three days he was drowsy, ataxic and his skin retained the chlorotic hue.

For nearly a fortnight his breathe, faeces and skin smelt of the oil and it was a clear fortnight before he felt really well again.

Case Citation: Kirkness WR (1910) Poisoning by oil of eucalyptus. Br Med J, 1: 261.

3) In 1906, Myott reported that, An adult male took approximately 25 mL of eucalyptus oil.

Within two hours he was dazed and friends successfully induced vomiting. Four hours after ingestion he was cyanosed with laboured breathing, foam in the mouth, congestion, rhonchi and moist rales throughout both lungs.

He was given oxygen with a stimulant and five to six hours later was restored enough to answer questions.

However 13 hours after ingestion he complained of difficulty and pain in drawing his breathe.

Breathing became more rapid and laboured, the pulse quick and thready and he died forty hours after taking the oil.

Presumably death was due to bronchopneumonia.

Case Citation: Myott MB (1906) Case of eucalyptus poisoning. Br Med J, 1: 558.

4) In 1965, Gurr et al., reported that, an adult who ingested 120 mL to 220 mL had severe poisoning and was successfully treated with mannitol, haemodialysis and peritoneal dialysis.

Case Citation: Gurr RW & Scroggie JG (1965) Eucalyptus oil poisoning treated by dialysis and mannitol infusion. Aust Ann Med, 4:238-249.

5) In 1953, Craig et al., reported that, a 7 month old boy was offered a teaspoonful of eucalyptus oil.

He coughed, choked and some of the oil was spilled.

He was pale, collapsed with rapid shallow respirations and feeble pulse 25 minutes later.

Limbs were flaccid, pupils pin-point, rhonchi being heard at both bases.

His stomach was washed out and three hours later he was showing spontaneous movement.

At 24 hours his general state was good.

The odour stayed on his breath for 72 hours.

This case is mentioned because it is often the source of the quote that as little as 1 mL can cause transient coma in an infant.

From the history this may or may not be the case but is hardly certain.

Case Citation: Craig JD (1953) Poisoning by the volatile oils in childhood. Arch Dis Child, 28: 475-483.

6) In 1953, Craig et al., reported that, a six year old boy took 4 mL to 5 mL of eucalyptus oil and within two hours severe vomiting had set in. Five hours later he was semi-comatose. There was no cough and breathing was shallow. After approximately eight hours the heavy comatose condition appeared to pass off.

He slept well but beyond being tired the next day was quite well.

The breathe smelt of eucalyptus oil for three days.

In summary the poisoning manifest itself as gastrointestinal irritation and cerebral paresis (Foggie, 1911).

Case Citation: Foggie WE (1911) Eucalyptus oil poisoning. Br Med J, 1: 359-360.

7) In 1893, Neale A et al., reported that, a 10 year old boy took approximately 15 mL of eucalyptus oil.

In a few minutes he was gasping for air and vomited heavily.

He breathed well for about an hour when the struggle for air increased until his death 15 hours after ingestion of the oil.

He spoke rationally several times up to within an hour of death.

There was only one vomit.

Case Citation: Neale A (1893) Case of death following blue gum (eucalyptus Globulus) oil. Aust Med Gazette, 12: 115-116.

8) In 1980, Patel S et al., reported that, a 3 year old boy took 10 mL of eucalyptus oil.

Within 30 minutes he was deeply comatose and his breath smelt strongly of eucalyptus.

Pupils were constricted, muscle tone markedly reduced and tendon reflexes could not be elicited.

Respirations were shallow and irregular. Blood pressure was 75/40 mmHg. Respiratory rate, blood pressure and pulse returned to normal after two and a half hours.

After five hours consciousness had gradually been regained and by 24 hours physical examination was normal apart from a faint smell of eucalyptus on the breathe.

Case Citation: Patel S & Wiggins J (1980) Eucalyptus oil poisoning. Arch Dis Child, 55: 405-406.

9) In 1909, Atkinson TR et al., reported that, a 6 year old was given approximately 15 mL of eucalyptus oil and experienced only slight drowsiness.

Case Citation: Atkinson TR (1909) Eucalyptus oil. Br Med J, 2: 1656.

SAFE DOSAGE

The safe adult dosage of eucalyptus oil as an internal medicine is quoted as 0.06ml to 0.2 ml.

Oral therapeutic doses of eucalyptus oil for adults are 0.05 to 0.2 ml, equivalent to 46 to 184 mg eucalyptol, and 0.3 – 0.6 g eucalyptus oil/day.

Maximum concentrations of eucalyptol in cosmetic products have been reported to be 0.4% in soap, 0.04% in detergents, 0.1% in creams and lotions and 1.6% in perfume.

Ref: Martindale W. The extra pharmacopoeia. 27th ed. London: Pharmaceutical Press, 1977.

CASE FATALITY

Death in adults has occurred after 4 or 5 ml, and is usual after 30 ml.

Citation: MacPherson J. The toxicology of eucalyptus oil. Med J Aust 1925; ii: 108-10.

RECOVERY RATE

Recovery however, has been reported after the ingestion of 120 to 220 ml.

The toxic effects of ingestion of this toxic, volatile hydrocarbon are rapid in onset and extensive.

They include a burning sensation in the mouth and throat, abdominal pain, and spontaneous vomiting which may be delayed up to 4 hours after ingestion.

Respiratory problems include bronchospasm and tachypnoea, with dangerous respiratory depression following severe intoxication.

Central nervous system involvement includes diminution or loss of reflexes, and depression of consciousness which may progress to coma.

Convulsions are rare in the adult but may be prominent in the child.

Direct nephrotoxicity may follow the ingestion of large volumes and cutaneous manifestations have been described.

Although the use of eucalyptus oil is becoming less fashionable, the hazards of its ingestion remain, particularly in the child.

Our case compilation serves as a reminder of the severe toxicity of this substance, illustrating the rapid onset of its severe respiratory and central nervous system effects.

POSTMORTEM FINDINGS

In one reported by Lewin(1897), a boy of 10, after taking 15 grams, suffered from vomiting, pallor of the lips, rapid weak pulse, sighing respiration, and air hunger, and died in fifteen minutes.

At the post-mortem examination, blood was found in the pleural cavity.

Citation: Lewin, Lehrbuch der Toxikologie, 2te Aufl.,1897.

NEPHROPATHY

Eucalyptol is widely distributed in plants.

The main food sources are eucalyptus oil (up to 80% eucalyptol), the herbs and spices mugwort, sweet basil, rosemary, sage and cardamom and their essential oils.

As part of a series of short-term studies on peppermint oil constituents for their possible induction of the encephalopathy found with peppermint oil, 1,8-cineole and l-limonene were studied.

1,8-Cineole and l-limonene both induced accumulation of protein droplets containing alpha 2 mu-globulin in proximal tubular epithelial cells in male rats.

These results by Kristiansen et al (1995) suggest that both 1,8-cineole and l-limonene possibly belong to the group of chemicals characterized by their induction of excessive alpha 2 mu-globulin accumulation.

Kristiansen E, Madsen C. Induction of protein droplet (alpha 2 mu-globulin) nephropathy in male rats after short term dosage with 1, 8-Cineole and l-limonene. Toxicol. Lett. 1995;80(1-3):147-52.

ANOTHER FATAL CASE

In a case of Myott's (1906), a man of 34, after tag 4 drachms became soon dazed and later unconscious.

The pulse became quick and the breathing laboured.

The physical signs pointed to congestion throughout both lungs.

He rallied a little, but died within forty hours after taking the oil.

The post-mortem examination showed inter alia reddening of the trachea and bronchi.

Citation: Myott, EC. BRITISH MEDICAL JOURNAL, i, 1906. p. 558.

MANAGING TOXICITY

The management of eucalyptus oil poisoning is mainly supportive.

Attempts to induce vomiting in the child should be avoided and the possibility of vomiting and aspiration of oil implies that gastric lavage should be performed with great care, a cuffed endotracheal tube being inserted in the presence of central nervous system depression.

Urinary output should be carefully monitored, particularly when hypotension is present or if large volumes of oil have been ingested.

In severe poisoning, peritoneal or haemodialysis is of value.

Ref: Spoerke DG, Vandenberg SA, Smolinske SC, Kulg K, Rumach BH. Eucalyptus oil: 14 cases of exposure. Vet Hum Toxicol. 1989;31:166–8.

SYSTEMIC TOXICITY

Oil of eucalyptus is a toxic substance capable of producing severe cardio-vascular, respiratory and central nervous system manifestations after ingestion by an adult of as little as 4 ml.

The literature describing this substance as a poison is reviewed, and a case of severe intoxication with prolonged coma is reported by Gurr RW et al (1965).

An adult who ingested 120 mL to 220 mL had severe poisoning and was successfully treated with mannitol, haemodialysis and peritoneal dialysis.

Successful management of this case included the use of mannitol, hemodialysis and peritoneal dialysis, and the contribution of these measures to the treatment of poisoning is discussed.

The effective removal of eucalyptol by dialysis suggests the application of this form of therapy to poisoning by other volatile oils.

Gurr RW & Scroggie JG (1965) Eucalyptus oil poisoning treated by dialysis and mannitol infusion. Aust Ann Med, 4: 238-249.

FIRST-AID MEASURES AND MANAGEMENT PRINCIPLES

First-aid measures. Avoid milk. All ingestions require medical assessment.

Stabilize patient by providing basic life support (i.e., airway, breathing and circulation).

Management is mainly symptomatic and supportive.

The main risk is aspiration because the principle toxic effects are vomiting and depression of conscious state.

Therefore, aggressive gastrointestinal decontamination without airway protection may in itself be harmful.

Attempts to induce vomiting must be avoided.

The best option for treating minor or moderate poisoning is close observation.

Asymptomatic patients should be observed for six hours.

If respiratory manifestations develop after ingestion, aspiration may have occurred.

An initial chest examination (including chest x-ray) is indicated.

If no abnormalities are detected on initial chest examination, repeat six hours after ingestion.

Careful gastric lavage and instillation of activated charcoal or colonic washout solution should only be attempted under general anaesthesia with endotracheal intubation.

DOES EUCALYPTUS OIL KILL CORONA VIRUS?

Effectivity of eucalyptol on curing covid illness is still under research, but its aroma & its flavored lozenges were very helpful in relieving the dry cough during corona pandemic.

LET'S SOLVE AN INTOXICATING RIDDLE
FOR "GUMS TO SAVE GUMS" SIR
Chewing Gums do save Gums of Teeth from microbial infections

DOES EUCALYPTUS OIL KILL MICROBES?

Laboratory studies later showed that eucalyptus oil contains substances that kill bacteria.

It also may kill some viruses and fungi.

Studies in animals and test tubes show that eucalyptus oil acts as an expectorant, meaning it helps coughs by loosening phlegm.

ITS STATUARY WARNING- DON'T MISUSE ZAI LEE TALL & THROW ABOUT

zai lee tall= Xy-li-tol= Xylitol

Chewing gums are misused after being chewed, placed on chairs, hair of people's backside or on pets, thus the sticky gum becomes a nuisance for getting rid off.

IS CHEWING GUM HARMFUL TO THE ENVIRONMENT?

Whether it's being used as a mid-day breath refresher or on the playground to see who can blow the biggest bubble—chewing gum is a daily habit for many people.

But what happens when you're done chewing it?

80–90% of chewing gum is not disposed of properly and it's the second most common form of litter after cigarette butts.

Chewing gum is made from polymers which are synthetic plastics that do not biodegrade.

When it's tossed on the sidewalk, there it sits until it's removed which can be a costly, time consuming process. Littered gum can also make it's way into the food chain.

It has been found in fish where it can accumulate toxins over time.

Sustainable chewing gums have been produced.

These gums are natural, biodegradable substances. Cities are also implementing gum receptacles to cut down on waste.

In a six month period these trash cans cut down on littered gum by 72%.

Next time you get ready to toss your gum, consider aiming for a trash can instead of the side walk.

Citation: https://www.custommade.com/blog/sustainable-gum/

trash can instead of the side walk.

Citation: https://www.custommade.com/blog/sustainable-gum/

AS IF I WAS LIKE A CHILDREN'S SUGARY BUBBLE CHEWING GUM TO HER

TEENS CHEW MY GUM &
BLOW BUBBLE TO SHOW
ME IN SELFIE POUT

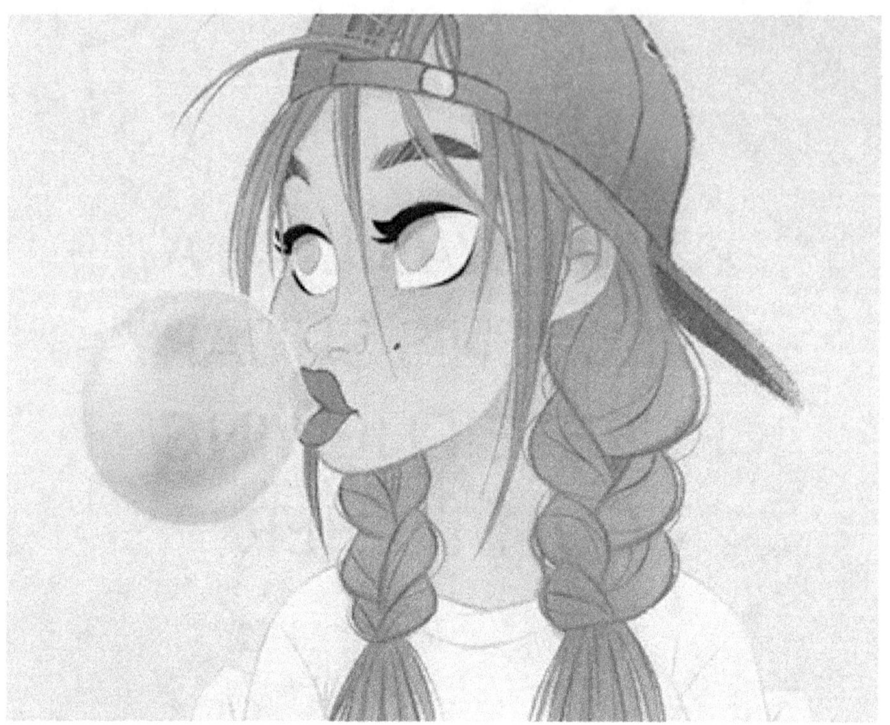

MASTICATING WELL, FOUND ME TASTELESS AFTER ENJOYING MY FLAVOR

Chewing gums are flavored with sweetness, but becomes tasteless after chewing well with molars & premolars, just like the rumination done by herbivores.

I HOLD THE GUINEA'S RECORD AS WORLD'S TALLEST ANGIOSPERM STOUT

The tallest living tree overall is not an angiosperm but a gymnosperm (vascular plants that lack flowers and fruit): the superlative specimen of Sequoia sempervirens, nicknamed Hyperion, is located in Redwood National Park in California, USA.

The coast redwood, a type of conifer known for its lofty stature, was discovered by Chris Atkins and Michael Taylor (both USA) on 25 August 2006 and, as of 2019, it stands 116.07 m (380 ft 9.7 in) tall.

The world's tallest angiosperm is currently an individual of Australian mountain ash, or swamp gum (Eucalyptus regnans) known as Centurion.

The Centurion, When initially climbed in 2009, the height was 99.60 m (326 ft 9.3 in) tall - 100.31 m (329 ft 1.2 in) to the low point of ground and 98.89 m (324 ft 5.3 in) to high point of ground. The most recent confirmed tape drop height was 99.82 m (327 ft 5.9 in), measured in 2014 by Steve Sillett. Ground-based measurements suggest that the tree had surpassed 100 m (328 ft) by 2018. The devastating 2019 Tasmanian bushfires killed many of Tasmania's largest trees, and the base of Centurion was moderately burned, although the treetop was initially still alive. In 2014, the tree had an estimated aboveground dry mass of 122 metric tonnes (135 US tons) and 541 kg (1,193 lb) dry mass of foliage.

Globally, eucalypts are also the world's tallest planted trees. Direct tape-drop has confirmed an 82.25-m-tall (269-ft 10.2-in) E. regnans near Dunedin, New Zealand (measured in 2018), a 79-m (259-ft 2.2-in) E. saligna near Polokwane, South Africa (measured in 2013) and a 72.9-m (239-ft 2.0-in) E. diversicolor near Coimbra, Portugal (measured in 2015).

Ref: Tallest flowering plant (angiosperm) https://www.guinnessworldrecords.com/world-records/572236-tallest-flowering-plant-angiosperm

DOUBLE MINT
CENTER FRESH PINK
BUBBLE YOU CALL
IIPPED US TWEET

You-call-lipped-us= Eu-cal-lypt-us- Eucalyptus (homophonic word sounds similar)

Double mint, Center fresh & Pink bubble are the brand names of commercial chewing gums derived from eucalyptus tree

BLOSSOMED, PETAL-LESS, CLOSED CUPPED FLOWERS BLOOM IN SPROUT

Eucalyptus Flowers Have No Petals

DO EUCALYPTUS TREES BLOOM?

From a distance, the flowers on most species of eucalyptus trees look like fluffy bursts of color, kind of like a dandelion flower gone to seed.

Get closer and you'll see why.

These breathtaking blossoms have no petals.

WHAT TIME OF YEAR DO GUM TREES FLOWER?

Flowering season: It flowers from December to January

The Red Gum tree blossoms every second year, usually the same year as Yellow Box, and concurrently with it.

The entire "bloom" consists of hundreds of stamens emerging from a central cone-like bud.

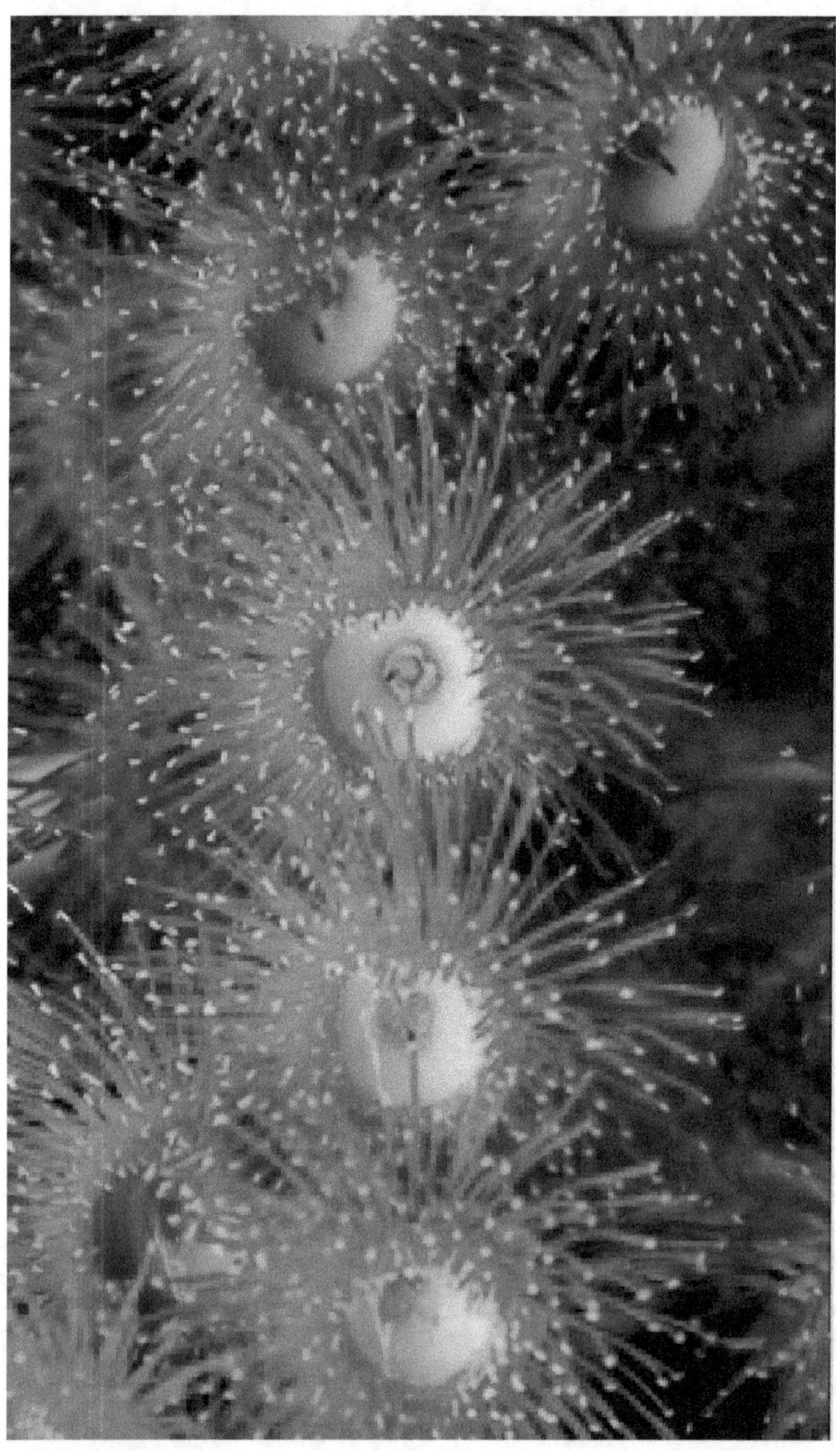

Figure 8. Eucalyptus Red Gum tree blooms

FERTILE FLUFFY HAIRED STAMENS SCENTS COUGH LOZENGES HONEY SWEET

They come in a range of colors including white, bright red, vibrant orange, deep pink, and lime green.

The abundance of stamens translates to an abundance of pollen.

And, eucalyptus trees can use as much pollen as possible.

They have few natural pollinators because of high concentrations of cineole.

Most often, eucalyptus trees count on the multitude of stamens for self-pollination.

COUGH LOZENGES:

CURRENT REGULATORY STATUS

Eucalyptol has been regarded as GRAS (generally recognised as safe) by FEMA (1965) and is approved by the US Food and Drug Administration (FDA) for food use.

The FDA advisory review panels on over-the-counter drugs have concluded that eucalyptol is safe for a variety of products, such as lozenges taken every 0.5 - 1 hr at 0.2 – 15 mg or taken every 2 hrs at 1 – 30 mg of eucalyptol (FDA, 1976 – 1990).

Highest exposure from food is likely to arise from hard (cough) candy in which up to about 130 mg eucalyptol/kg or about 2000 mg eucalyptus oil/kg have been reported to be used (Fenaroli, 1995).

Consumption of 10 g of hard candy containing 2000 mg eucalyptus oil/kg would result in an intake of up to 16 mg of eucalyptol, equivalent to 0.27 mg/kg bw for an adult of 60 kg.

Eucalyptol - European Commission(2000) - europa.eu https:// ec.europa.eu/food/sites/food/files/safety/docs/sci-com_scf_out126_en.pdf

FOR VENOMOUS WASPS & HONEYBEES TO BUZZ SPURIOUS BLACK ABOUT

Spurious black is the slang name of eucalyptus tree in Australia

Australia's crowning woodland glory has only survived long enough to grow so tall by chance.

Most of the surrounding area has been heavily logged, and forest fires regularly sweep through these remote regions.

A bushfire in February 2019 came close to ending it all, badly charring Centurion's base despite heroic efforts to save the tree from harm.

But it's not all bad news. Eucalyptus trees have evolved along-side the ever-present threat of fire, and Centurion remains stable and healthy, even with its blackened trunk, thus known as Spurious black.

SQUARE STEMS AND UNCOMMON LEAF FORMATIONS

Small branches of eucalyptus trees and shrubs are popular in flower arrangements. Why?

In part because of their sturdiness and the visual appeal of their leaf formation.

While most trees have round stems, eucalyptus stems are closer to the square.

The natural advantage of this shape is unclear, but that doesn't detract from its beauty.

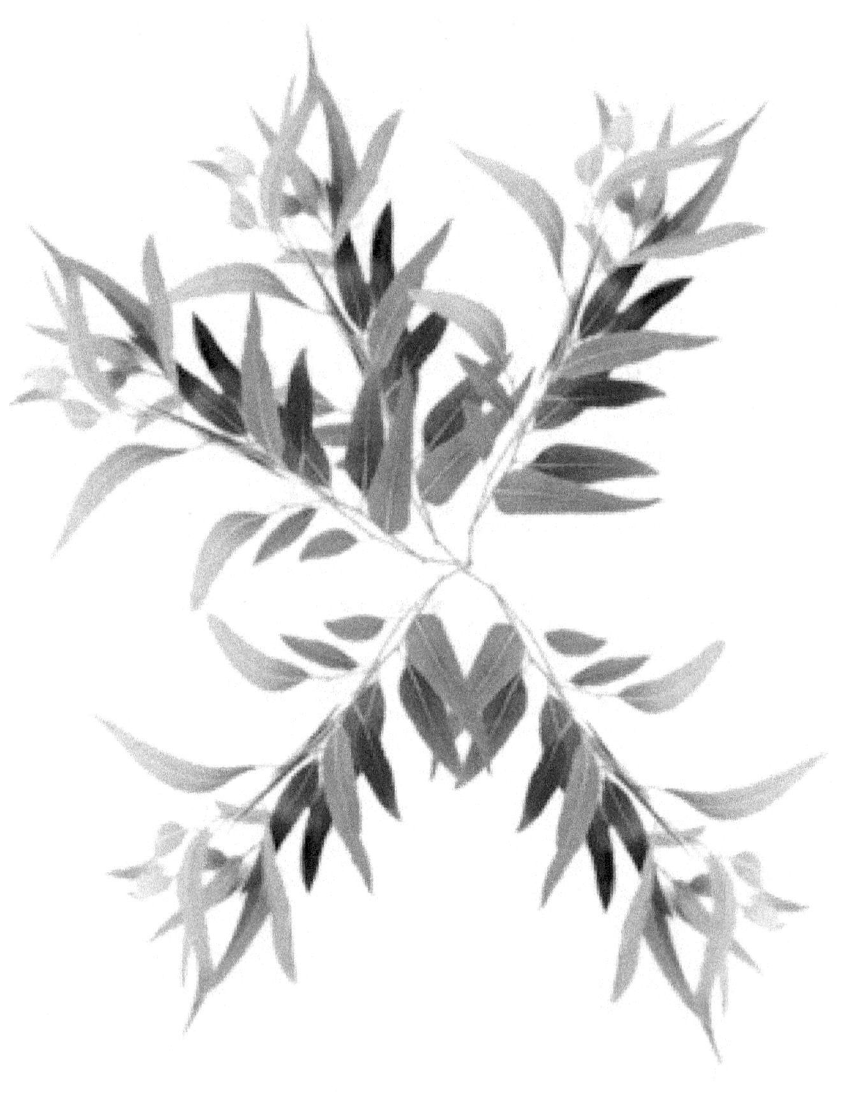

What also makes the stems and branches of eucalyptus trees compelling is the way the leaves grow.

They grow in pairs on opposite sides of the stem.

But the neighboring pairs of leaves are at right angles to each other.

So a pattern of A-C, B-D, A-C, B-D, etc. emerges where A, B, C, and D are the four sides of the stem.

NILGIRIS TREE BARK MAKE WHITENED VICKS VAPORUB ON CHEST TO MEET

The eucalyptus oil was also called 'Nilgiri Taila' because of its area of cultivation, in India.

The oil was widely extracted in the hills of OOTY = Udagamand (Nilgiris, South India).

Located 89 kms from Coimbatore, Ooty deservedly earns its reputation as the 'Queen of Hill Stations' for its extensive tea plantations, lakes and other natural splendors.

WHAT IS THE CONTENTS OF CHEST VAPORUBS?

Eucalyptus derived Vaporubs Contain

- Camphor 5.26%,
- Menthol 2.82%, Thymol 0.09%,
- Oil of Eucalyptus 6%,
- Nutmeg 0.69%,
- Cedar Leaf 0.44%
- Turpentine 4.68%,
- Petroleum jelly 10%.

CHEST VAPORUB DERMAL TOXICITY TO TODDLER

Toddler girl presented to A&E with second seizure after her mother applied a camphor chest rub too often to the child's chest, back, and head – every hour for 10 hours – to treat cold symptoms.

Flaman Z, Pellechia-Clarke S, Bailey B, McGuigan M. Unintentional exposure of young children to camphor and eucalyptus oils. Paediatr Child Health. 2001;6(2):80-83. doi:10.1093/pch/6.2.80

CHEST VAPORUB ORAL TOXICITY TO TODDLER

A 19-month-old female (10.7 kg) ate approximately 50 mL of Vicks VapoRub ointment.

One hour later she had a seizure at home and appeared lethargic afterwards.

Her parent did not take her to an acute care hospital until 4 h after exposure.

On arrival at the emergency department, the toddler was asymptomatic.

She remained seizure-free and was discharged 24 h after admission.

Flaman Z, Pellechia-Clarke S, Bailey B, McGuigan M. Unintentional exposure of young children to camphor and eucalyptus oils. Paediatr Child Health. 2001;6(2):80-83. doi:10.1093/pch/6.2.80

KOALA BEARS GATHER GUM-NUTS FROM US TO SING A SONG THROUGH OUT

koala bears love munching their leaves, that is. And the male Koala sings in their low pitch voice, as it clears the throat.

Didgeridoos are a long, trumpet-like instrument with a deep history among the Indigenous people of Australia.

Traditionally, it's played during ceremonial dancing and singing.

Today, it's also played for recreation.

But no matter why it's played, many who know about these things contend that the best didgeridoos are made from eucalyptus wood.

Traditional production involves finding a tree trunk or major branch that's been hollowed out by termites.

The trunk or limb is then cut down, cleaned inside, and stripped of its bark.

The hardness of eucalyptus wood helps create pleasing acoustics when played.

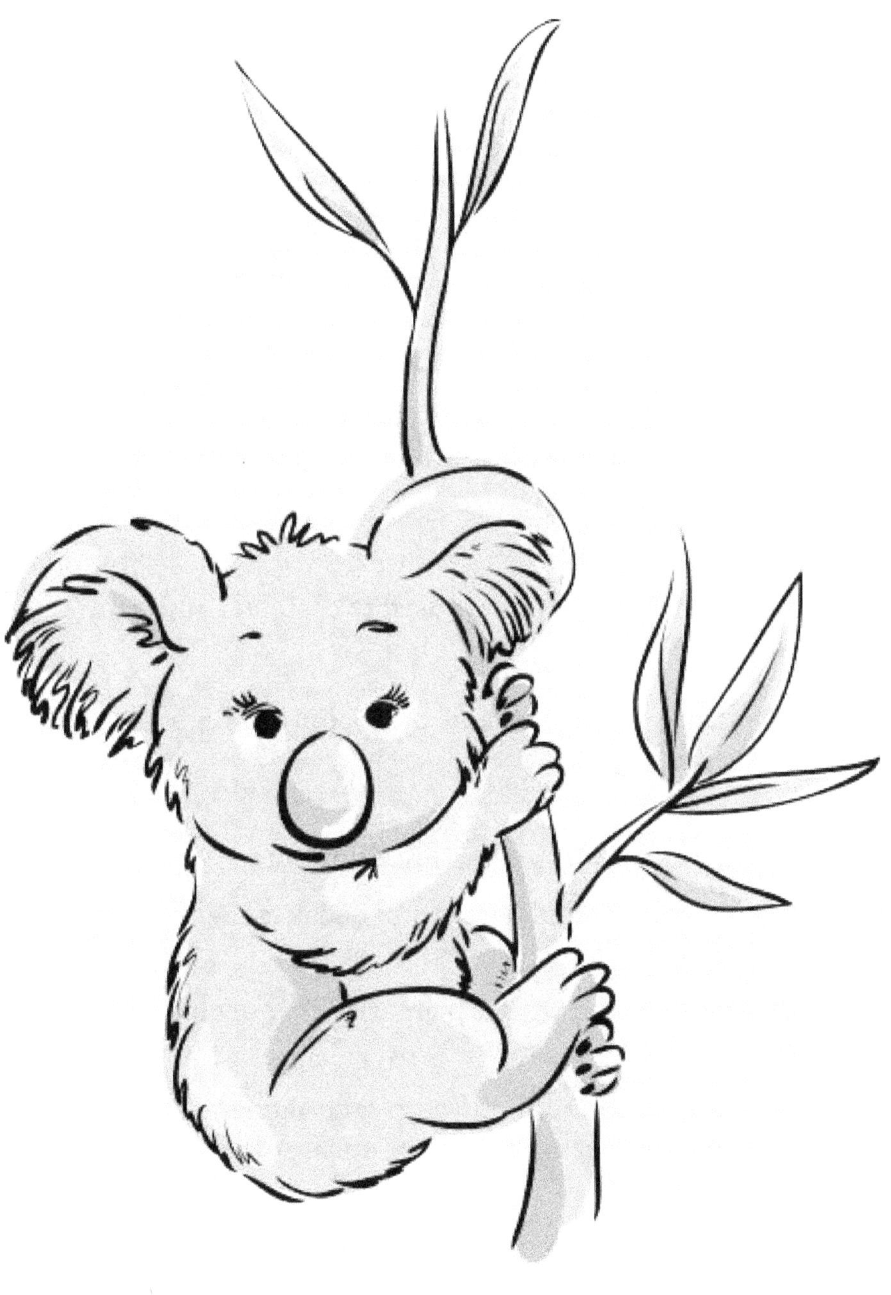

CINEOLE: THE SECRET INGREDIENT

Eucalyptus essential oil has been used in Indigenous Australian medicine as an antibacterial and anti-fungal agent for centuries.

In India's Ayurvedic medicine, it's often used in the treatment of respiratory ailments.

In 17th century England, it was used to disinfecting hospitals.

Why?

Because eucalyptus leaves and bark contain high concentrations of cineole.

Cineole is a colorless, liquid organic compound.

It's sometimes also called eucalyptol because there's so much of it in eucalyptus trees and shrubs.

The fragrance of eucalyptus is primarily that of cineole.

We don't want to sound like a high school chemistry tutorial, so let's simply say that cineole is the eucalyptus' secret weapon against predators.

Only the koala bear, ring-tail possum, and a few insects can eat eucalyptus leaves and bark.

No other creature, including humans, can withstand the high levels of cineole.

In fact, in high concentrations, it's toxic.

That's why it makes an effective and natural insect repellent.

Clinical research has proven the anti-bacterial, antiseptic, and anti-fungal properties of cineole.

Using eucalyptus essential oil in topical wound treatment, skincare, and other disinfecting applications makes sense.

HIGH RISK FOR KIDS TO CHOKE, IF THEY SLEPT & ASPIRATE GUMS THEY EAT

Foreign body aspiration is a major cause of morbidity and mortality in children.

Nearly 80% of choking events occur in infants younger than 3 years.

Nineteen percent of choking events are caused by candy or gum, neither of which is subject to regulation by the Federal Hazardous Substances Act.

The American Academy of Pediatrics states that gum should not be given to children who are "too young to understand that they shouldn't swallow it."

However, there are no formal recommendations regarding specific age restrictions in India.

The majority of airway foreign bodies are found in the proximal bronchial tree.

A delay in presentation is associated with increased risk for complications such as pulmonary inflammation, recurrent pneumonia, and bronchiectasis.

As a result, timely evaluation and management are essential.

Rigid bronchoscopy is considered the standard of care for evaluation and management of foreign body aspiration.

Chewing gum aspiration can present a particular dilemma, in that fragments of gum may not be easily extracted.

MAY STUCK THE BLUE GUMSTICK INTO AIRWAY INSTEAD OF SPITTING IT OUT

Gumstick is the brand name of one of the chewing gums derived from eucalyptus.

CHEWING GUM CHOKING

Therapeutic Challenges after Chewing Gum Aspiration in a Toddler: A Case Report

Matthew FA, et al.(2106) reported an interesting case of 19-month-old previously healthy boy presented to an outside emergency department with 4 days of cough and progressively worsening respiratory distress.

Initial physical examination findings revealed tachypnea, decreased aeration of the lungs, and wheezing, for which the patient received an inhaled bronchodilator, a corticosteroid, and supplemental oxygen.

He was also given an intravenous dose of ceftriaxone after a chest radiograph showed near-complete opacification of the left hemithorax.

Despite those interventions, he required initiation of noninvasive positive pressure ventilation and was transferred to our tertiary care center for further management.

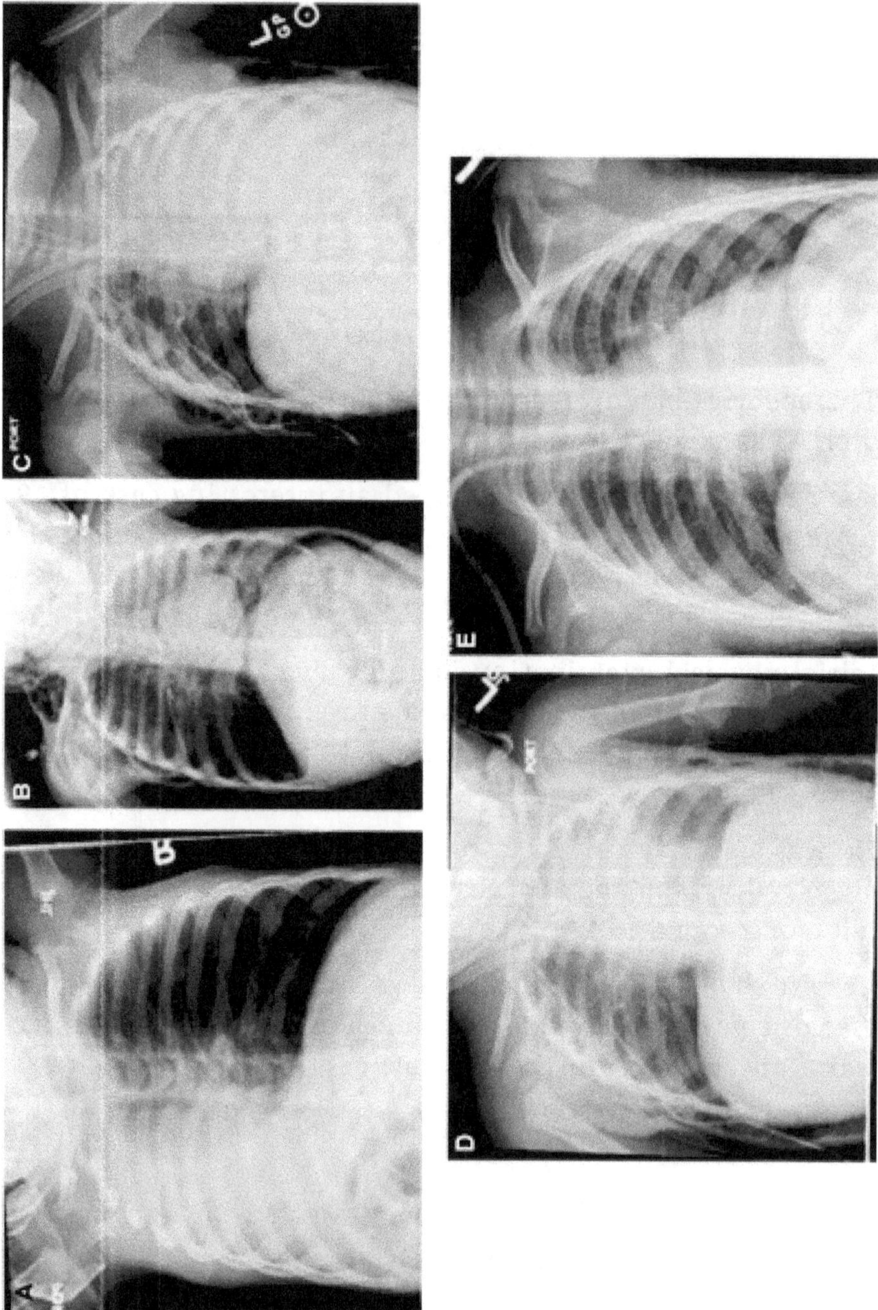

Figure 9. Chewing Gum Aspiration in a Toddler (A) Initial X-ray (posterior-anterior) with right-sided hyperinflation and tracheal deviation. (B) After first bronchoscopy. Note significant subcutaneous emphysema. (C) Worsening left-sided

opacities despite high peak pressures. (D) Immediately after ice-cold saline lavage. (E) Near-complete resolution before discharge. Image source: Matthew FA, et al. (2016) Annals of the American Thoracic Society. 13988-990.

On arrival, a repeat chest radiograph confirmed complete opacification of the left hemithorax and also demonstrated hyperexpansion of the right lung with deviation of the trachea to the left.

A detailed history revealed that the patient had been given chewing gum on several occasions in the recent past.

Because of concern for chewing gum aspiration, he was taken to the operating room for bronchoscopic foreign body extraction.

While under anesthesia, the patient was notably difficult to ventilate, showing wide swings in pulmonary compliance and arterial oxygen saturation.

Rigid bronchoscopy revealed diffusely inflamed airways.

Multiple gum fragments were located in the left bronchial tree.

Larger fragments of foreign material were extracted using a forceps, but flexible bronchoscopy was unsuccessful in the removal of smaller fragments from distal airways.

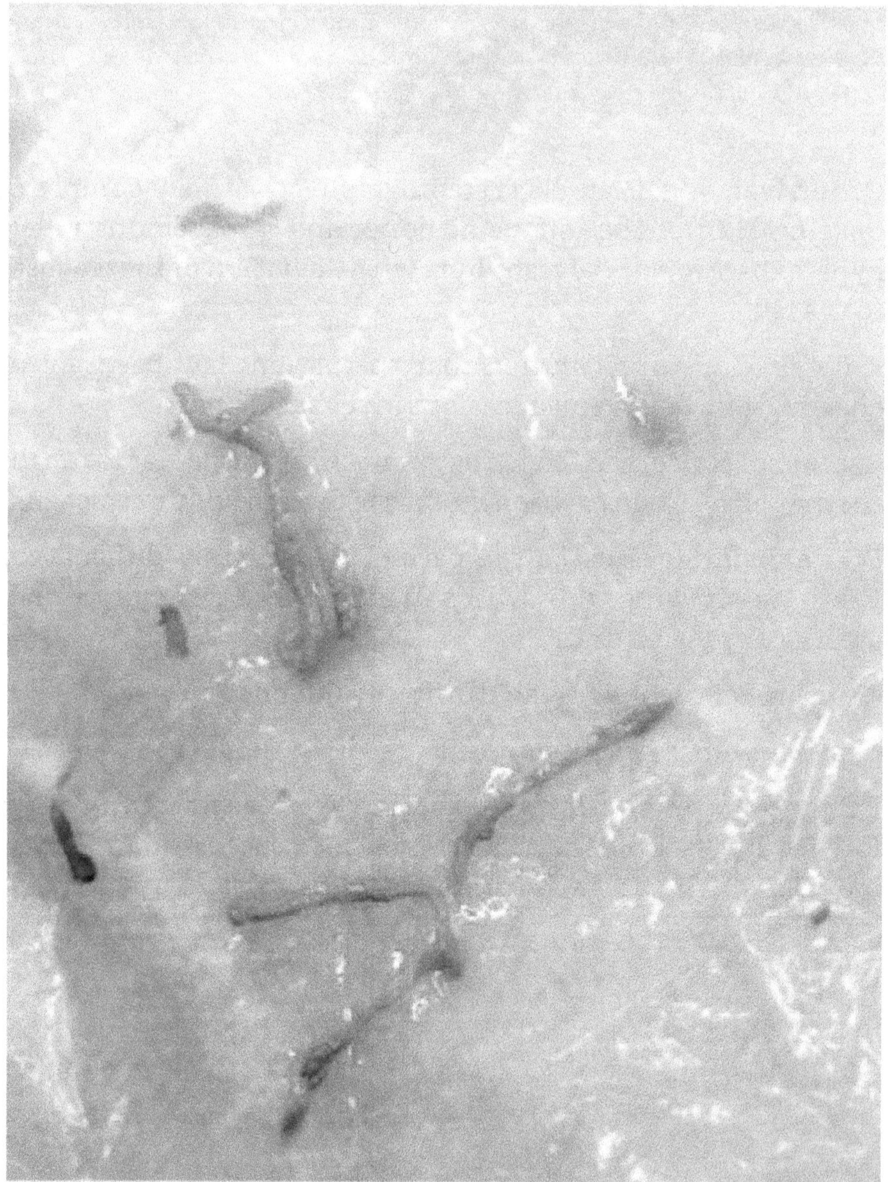

Figure 10. Multiple large chewing gum casts after forceps extraction in a Toddler. Image source: Matthew FA, et al. (2016) Annals of the American Thoracic Society. 13988-990.

After the procedure, patient could not maintain adequate ventilation despite high peak pulmonary pressures of 60–90 mm Hg.

He developed a right-sided pneumothorax with mediastinal and subcutaneous emphysema and was emergently placed on extracorporeal membrane oxygenation (ECMO).

One day later, he developed a nonhemorrhagic stroke in the distribution of the right middle cerebral artery.

Given the urgent need for ECMO decannulation, an emergent bronchoscopy was requested to assist in further removal of foreign body material.

Bedside reexamination with a flexible bronchoscope revealed a number of small chewing gum fragments throughout the left bronchial tree.

In an attempt to remove the remaining gum fragments, several aliquots of ice-cold saline were instilled into the lobar bronchi of the left lung, which yielded substantial return of foreign material upon suctioning.

Before completion of the procedure, 10 ml hypertonic sodium bicarbonate was instilled into the left lung lobar bronchi in an attempt to dissolve the remaining gum fragments.

This technique did not yield any consequential further return of gum fragments.

In less than 1 hour, there was remarkable improvement in ventilation parameters and aeration of the left lung.

Patient was decannulated from ECMO circuitry later that day and went on to make a full recovery.

Chest radiographic findings were normal shortly before hospital discharge.

This case highlights therapeutic challenges that may be encountered in the management of chewing gum aspiration.

Removal of gum fragments distributed throughout proximal

and distal airways of our patient required a coordinated multidisciplinary effort that included both rigid and flexible bronchoscopy.

CRYO: FREEZING CHEWING GUM HARDENS

The process of freezing chewing gum hardens the material.

This well-known effect has long been applied to remove tightly adherent gum from household surfaces.

In above case, ice-cold saline lavage facilitated removal of small gum fragments that eluded extraction from distal airways by conventional methods.

Previous reports have indicated that targeted cryotherapy can be effective in the removal of aspirated chewing gum.

Rubio E, Gupta P, Ie S, Boyd M. Cryoextraction: a novel approach to remove aspirated chewing gum. Ann Thorac Med 2013;8:58–59.

GUM STICKS

Sticking gums for gluing paper cuttings in school artwork are also derived from eucalyptus.

SUGAR GUM LEAVES THE SIGH A KNIGHED, TOXIC TO 24 GOATS ON FOUR FEET

Sigh A Knighed= Cy-anide

Many ruminants have faced cyanide poisoning, by eating especial variety of eucalyptus calocalyx leaves, rich in cyanogenic alkaloids, as self defense from ruminant predators.

Rumination is the habits of herbivore animals to keep chewing the grass for a long time in their mouth, especially goats, buffalo, cows & Horses.

Rumination is a method of mastication high fibre rich grasses & leaves, to first soak in saliva, to soften it, and then to chew by molars & premolars, to let it into fine pieces.

Chewing gums by humans simulate the habit of rumination, but it is not for nutrition, but just for keeping the mouth occupied into mastication.

Many gets confused to see someone chewing gum, that he is talking, when he is just maticating a chewing gum

CYANIDE POISONING OF GOATS FROM SUGAR GUMS

Fatal cyanide poisoning occurred in 24 of 50 Angora goats between two and 24 hours after eating leaves from a freshly felled sugar gum (Eucalyptus cladocalyx). In PM examination the blood failed to clot and was bright red. Chewed leaves of the tree comprised less than 5% of the total rumen contents, which had the typical "bitter almond" smell. Treatment of visibly affected goats with sodium nitrite and sodium thiosulphate intravenously, was followed by recovery of 26 goats within 24 hours. It is pointed out that free HCN in the rumen should be fixed by oral as well as intravenous treatment, which may need to be repeated because of continuing liberation of HCN in the rumen.

Webber JJ, Roycroft CR, Callinan JD (1985) Cyanide poisoning of goats from sugar gums (Eucalyptus cladocalyx). Aust Vet J 62(1):28.

MY LITTER IS LOT IN SO HUGE & HIGHLY FLAMMABLE TO GET ON FIRED SEAT

Litter of Gums & Gum tree

Litter of Chewing gums is 2nd highest in the world ranking, after the cigarette butts as 1st, as non-biodegradable health hazard.

Litter of Gum tree, in form of dry leaves, is potentially hazardous, as its flammable, due to rich content of combustible oil (eucalyptol).

I'M AUSTRALIAN FOREST FIRE HAZARD, BUSHFIRE MOUNTAIN ASH TO SNOUT

RAPID VAPORIZATION OF MY AROMA OILS RESULTS IN QUICK IGNITE TO LIT

These hardy plants have delightfully scented, volatile oil in all parts of the plant.

Thus the eucalyptus trees on hills are also known as Mountain Ash.

The tree sheds bark and dead leaves, which make a perfect pile of tinder under the tree too.

When the oils in the tree heat up, the plant releases flammable gas, which ignites into a fireball.

This accelerates the eucalyptus fire hazards in a region and discourages firefighting efforts.

The oil leaves a smoggy miasma hanging over the eucalyptus groves.

This gas is extremely flammable and the cause of many wild fires.

Read more at Gardening Know How: Eucalyptus

Fire Hazards: Are Eucalyptus Trees Flammable https://www.gardeningknowhow.com/ornamental/trees/eucalyptus/eucalyptus-fire-hazards.htm

THE SWAMP GUM FROM MY POINTED LEAVES, SICKLE-SHAPED STOUT

BUT I HAVE A SADDEST GUM OF SORROW,
TO SHARE WITH ALL OF U A BIT,
I GOT SO BLAMED BY AGREE CULTURE, FOR
SUCKING SOIL'S NUTRIENTS OUT

Eucalyptus Grows Super Fast, sucking soil's nutrients rapidly & deeply seated by its long roots, due to which the farmers avoid planting them near their farms.

One of the reasons it's an environment-friendly choice is the rate at which the trees grow.

Many varieties reach early maturity ten years after planting.

That's super-fast, compared to other hardwoods, which can take 18-25 years to reach early maturity.

Provided they have enough water and are in the right climate, eucalyptus trees are a renewable resource.

That's a remarkable and important fact for the sustainability of the flooring industry and for consumers who want to make better choices for the environment.

Whether you use eucalyptus trees for essential oils, didgeridoos, or flooring, you get value.

And in ten years, someone else can also enjoy the benefits of another eucalyptus tree.

SO BANNED TO CULTIVATE IN INDIA, BY HON'BLE COURT'S ORDER TO HIT

Protests about planting eucalyptus trees southeast of Bangkok rocked the Thai government in 1991, as villagers raided nurseries and ripped out seedlings.

Local people were objecting to government support for planting eucalyptus on public lands, especially because authorities intended to turn the trees into commercial pulp to feed the expanding international market for paper and newsprint.

BANNED TO CULTIVATE IN INDIA, AS PER HON'BLE COURT'S ORDER TO HIT

Ban took place about the same time in Karnataka High court (India) in 2017 order, after international groups, including the World Bank, collaborated with national and state agencies in covering thousands of hectares with quick-growing eucalyptus plantations.

Again, rural folk felt excluded.

In Spain and Portugal, farmers and others have also yanked seedlings out of the ground.

There, protesters characterized the multiplication of gridlike stands of these hardwoods as "capitalist" or "fascist," thus equating major plantings with rightwing politics during the Franco era.

Citation: Puntasen, "Political Economy of Eucalyptus"; Boland, "Australian Trees in Five Overseas Countries," p. 76; Environmental Defense Fund, "Failure of Social Forestry in Karnataka"; Montalbano, "'Fascist' Trees.

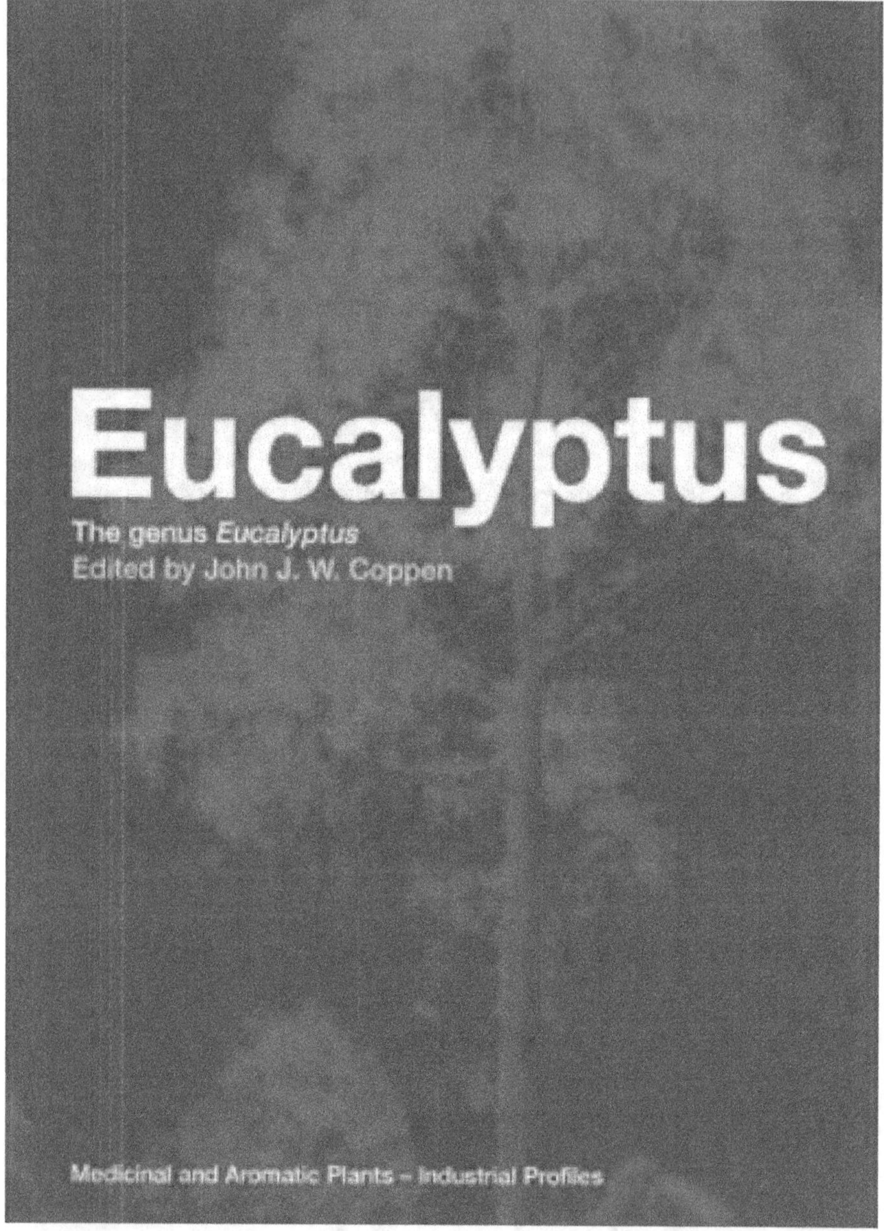

Figure 11. Eucalyptus: The Genus Eucalyptus (Medicinal and Aromatic Plants - Industrial Profiles) Coppen. John J.W. 2002. CRC Press

KOALA SONG

Koalas have an extra set of vocal cords outside the voice box that allow males to hit extremely low notes, researchers have discovered.

What kind of noise does a koala make?

Both male & female koalas can make types of bellowing calls, though it's usually made by males looking to attract a mate. They also make a variety of other sounds including snarls, squeaks and screams.

CHEWING GUMS OF BLUE, RED & WHITE

red gum tree– Eucalyptus camaldulensis

Blue gum tree –see– Eucalyptus globulus

sugar gum –see– Eucalyptus cladocalyx

Myers, Vanessa Richins. "Natural Chewing Gum History and Facts." ThoughtCo, Sep. 23, 2020, thoughtco.com/does-chewing-gum-come-from-gum-trees-3269782.

HOW TO IDENTIFY EUCALYPTUS

• Leaves: Carefully examine the leaves of the tree. Eucalyptus has protracted and pointed leaves with leathery texture and flat sides. A closer look at the leaves, especially with a magnifying glass, will give you the opportunity to see the oil-secreting glands throughout the leaves.

• Branches: Closely observe the branches of the tree. Adult eucalyptus leaves are sickle-shaped, which alternate on the branches on which they grow.

• Flowers: Look for flowers budding from the branches. Eucalyptus flowers look like closed cups before they bloom and when they open, there are no petals but fluffy hair, which are actually flower stamens.

• Fruit: Explore the flower stems to look for fruit growth. Looking like a small, woody capsule, eucalyptus fruit grows until it splits open and ejects seeds.

• Bark: Touch the bark to determine its texture, which is usually tough and flaky. In most of the species, there is seasonal shedding of the outermost bark layer.

The amount of litter dropped by eucalyptus is huge. Eucalyptus litter is highly flammable and a fire hazard. This is because of rapid vaporization of oils that results in rapid ignition.

CONTRIBUTORS:

1. Dr Yatin Mehta, Chairman, Anaesthesia, Critical Care, Emergency & Trauma care, Medanta-The Medicity, Gurugram
2. Dr P Venugopalan, Director, Emergency & Trauma care, MIMS, Calicut
3. Mr Santosh Kumar Verma, Senior Advocate, Rajasthan High Court
4. Dr Tariq Ali, Director, Critical Care, Medanta-The Medicity, Gurugram
5. Dr Praveen Aggarwal, Professor & Head, Department of Emergency Medicine, AIIMS, New Delhi
6. Dr Venkat Raghav, Professor & HOD, Forensic Medicine & toxicology, Bangalore Medical College, Bengaluru.
7. Dr Ajay Gangele, Professor, Forensic Medicine & Toxicology, DY Patil Medical college, Pune
8. Dr Krishnadutt Chavali, Professor, Forensic Medicine & Toxicology, AIIMS, Raipur
9. Dr SK Singhal, Professor &HOD, Forensic Medicine & Toxicology, Ananta Institute of Medical sciences and research center, Rajsamand (Rajasthan).
10. Dr Dhruv Chaudhary, Senior Professor & Head, Pulmonary & Critical Care Medicine, PGIMS, Rohtak
11. Dr Tejas Prajapati, Consultant Toxicologist, AMC MET Medical College, Ahmedabad, Gujarat
12. Dr Karen Harshita, Senior Resident, Forensic Medicine & Toxicology, Bangalore medical College and research institute, Bangalore
13. Dr Ajith Antony Senior Resident, Forensic Medicine & Toxicology, Goa
14. Dr Lishu Chaure, Senior Resident, Palamu Medical College,

Palamu Jharkhand.

15. Dr Somashekar Chandren, Assistant professor Forensic Medicine & Toxicology, AIMS, B G Nagara, Mandya, Karnataka

16. Dr Latif Johnson, Assistant professor, Forensic Medicine & Toxicology, Christain Medical College, Vellore

17. Dr Arjit Dey, Senior Resident, Forensic Medicine & Toxicology, AIIMS, Delhi

18. Dr Kashif Ali, Senior Resident, Forensic Medicine & Toxicology,

Jawaharlal Nehru Medical College, AMU, Aligarh (UP)

19. Dr. Sweta H Patel, Assistant Professor, Forensic Medicine & Toxicology, Pramukhswami Medical College, Karamsad. Dist. Anand, Gujarat.

20. Dr Suman K. Charawati, Scientist, Forensic Science Lab, Assam

21. Dr Walter Waz, Professor, Forensic Medicine & Toxicology, Mumbai

22. Dr Vatsal Pawnar, BAMS, Diploma in Cosmetology, Ayurvedic Cosmetologist, Gurugram

23. Dr Vidusha Vijay, Forensic Medicine & Toxicology Consultant, Columbia Asia Hospital Bangalore

24. R. R. Rajitha, Emergency Nursing officer, King Faisal Hospital, Riyadh, Saudi Arabia

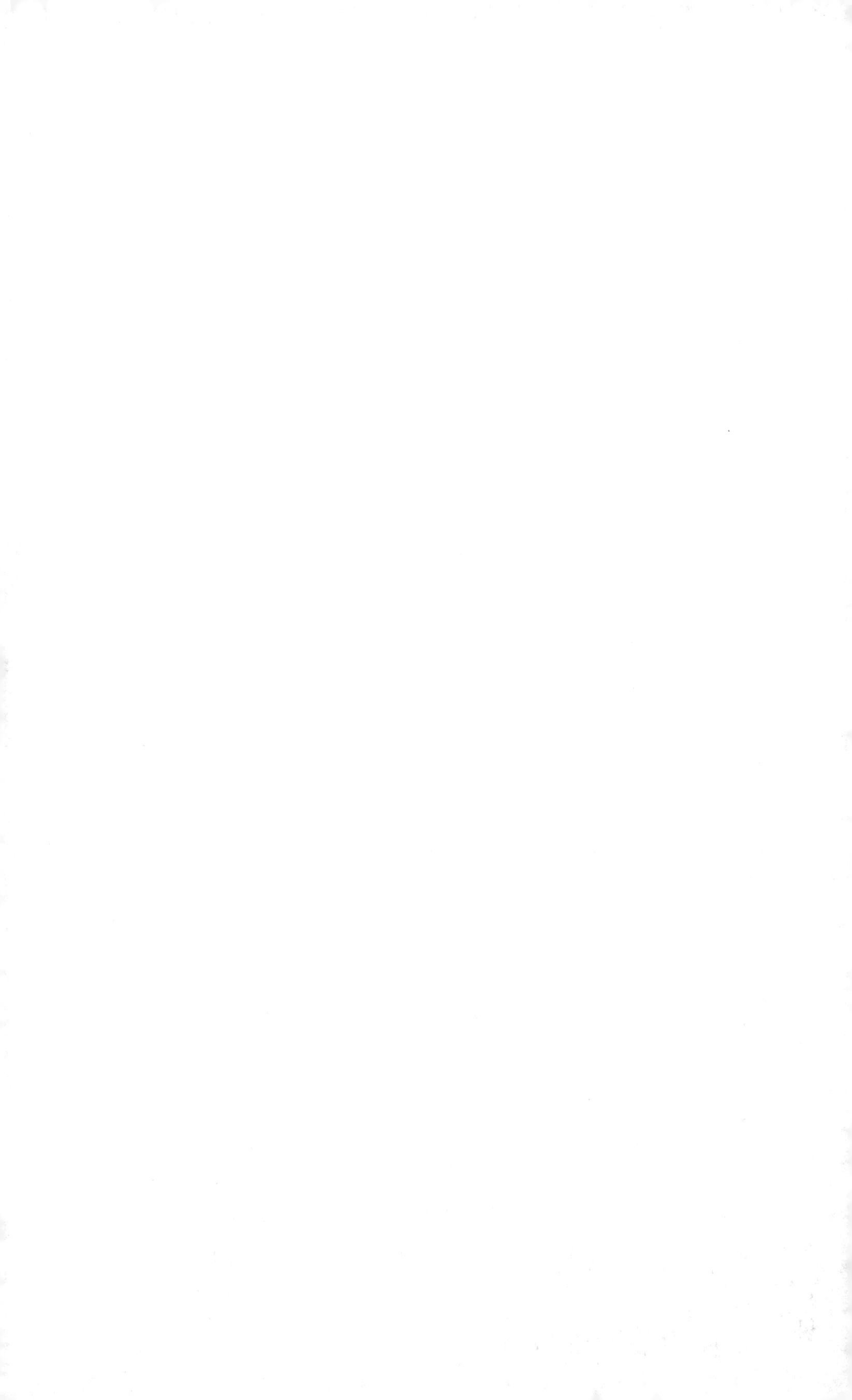